WHEN STRESS STRIKES . . .
LET KAVA HELP

FIND OUT ABOUT . . .

* The mental effects of kava . . . will you feel zoned out or mentally alert?

* How long it takes kava to work

* Important warnings about kava and drug interactions

* Your best bet for making kava taste better

* Kava with company or in cafés . . . how social is this herb?

* If kava can make you feel high

* Kava quality control—ways to ensure you get the potency you need

* Kava for depression, anxiety, PMS, menopausal symptoms, headache, muscle tightness, neck and shoulder pain . . .

and more!

KAVA
The Ultimate Guide to Nature's
Anti-Stress Herb

KAVA

The Ultimate Guide to Nature's Anti-Stress Herb

Maggie Greenwood-Robinson, Ph.D.

A Dell Book

Published by
Dell Publishing
a division of
Random House, Inc.
1540 Broadway
New York, New York 10036

ISBN: 0-440-23460-3

Design by Carol Russo

Printed in the United States of America
Published simultaneously in Canada

May 1999
10 9 8 7 6 5 4 3 2
OPM

To Jeffry with love

The suggestions for usage of kava and other supplements are not intended to replace medical advice or treatment by your physician or mental health counselor. All questions and concerns regarding your health and the treatment of stress, anxiety, depression, insomnia, and other medical conditions (including pregnancy and breast-feeding) should be directed toward your physician or mental health counselor. Long-term use of supplements is not recommended unless it is done under the guidance and supervision of a physician. Please consult your physician prior to supplementing with kava, herbs, and other supplements.

All reasonable attempts have been made to include the most recent and factual research and medical reports about kava and other supplements. However, there is no guarantee that future studies will not change the recommendations and information presented here.

The mention of specific products or brands in this book does not constitute an endorsement by either the author or the publisher.

Neither the publisher nor the author takes any responsibility for the possible consequences from any treatment, action, or application of medicine, herb, or preparation to any person reading or following the information in this book.

Acknowledgments

I gratefully thank the following people for their work and contributions to this book: Madeleine Morel, 2M Communications, Ltd.; Christine Zika, Dell Publishing; John Armstrong, vice president, Elixr Tea & Tonics; and Don Ansley, Better Living Products.

Contents

CHAPTER 1

The Wonder Herb
of the South Pacific

Imagine a natural remedy with the power to lift the stress and strain of everyday life . . . subdue anxiety . . . brighten a blue mood . . . and help you sleep like a baby at night.

Sound too good to be true?

Perhaps. Yet such a remedy really does exist! It's an herb called kava-kava (kava for short), and it's one of the most amazing nutritional supplements ever to hit the shelves. Grown on the islands of the South Pacific, kava is a veritable dream supplement, remarkable for its ability to treat stress, anxiety, depression, insomnia, and more. It is significant to note that kava's benefits have been verified by extensive research.

Kava produces a noticeable and pleasurable feeling of calm—without side effects or aftereffects. Virtually safe and nonaddictive in moderate doses, kava is fast becoming one of the hottest-selling herbs around, part of the $12.4 billion plus herb market worldwide. In 1998, consumers spent $50 million on kava alone!

Some experts feel kava is destined to be the biggest herbal supplement of all time because it offers a natural way to relieve stress—something everyone has, yet no one wants.

Clearly, kava is gaining runaway popularity, especially among the overworked of this generation, and decades of scientific research say it's just the antidote we need to unwind and de-stress.

IS KAVA A SUPPLEMENT OR A DRUG?

First and foremost, kava is an herb—one that has been approved by the United States Food and Drug Administration (FDA) as a dietary supplement. An herb is a plant, or a part of a plant, valued for its medicinal qualities, aroma, or taste. Herbs and herbal remedies have been used through the ages, in every culture and civilization. The Bible and other religious texts mention herbs to promote healing. Ancient civilizations such as the Chinese, Greek, and Roman practiced herbal medicine for centuries. Until the twentieth century, physicians routinely prescribed herbal-based medicines for their patients. In fact, your grandmother and great-grandmother probably relied on herbs to treat illnesses in their day.

Nearly 50 percent of all our modern drugs are derived from herbs or contain a chemical imitation of a plant compound. One of the best known is aspirin. In the early 1800s, its active ingredient, salicin, was isolated with white willow bark, an anti-inflammatory plant used for thousands of years, and eventually synthesized into a chemical imitation known to us as aspirin. Penicillin, the kingpin of all antibiotics, is a mold produced by a type of primitive plant known as a fungus. Digitalis, an important drug used to treat congestive heart failure, was discovered two hundred years ago from an ingredient in foxglove, a common garden flower grown in England. Quinidine, an important cardiac drug, and its relative, quinine, long used to treat malaria, both come from the bark of the Peruvian cinchona tree. Another bark-derived drug, taxol, now shows promise as a powerful cancer-fighting drug. And numerous drugs prescribed in Europe today contain extracts of kava. Even now pharmaceutical companies are scouring rain forests and other primitive locales to find native remedies and botanicals that may hold the cures for modern diseases.

RESURGENCE OF INTEREST IN HERBAL MEDICINE

Today there is a revival of tidal-wave proportions in the use of herbs to treat physical and mental disease. It is estimated that sixty million Americans now take herbs to help cure what ails them, from colds to allergies, from headaches to insomnia. And, according to the World Health Organization, 80 percent of the world's population uses herbs.

The reason for such popularity is that herbs work *with* your body's natural healing mechanisms, not against them. Many prescription medicines, on the other hand, can be quite toxic to the body and may tear down health rather than build it up. Over the years there have been many incidents in which approved pharmaceutical agents were yanked from the market because they had serious, sometimes fatal side effects. It is now estimated that accidental deaths from adverse reactions to prescription drugs are the fourth leading cause of death in the United States, claiming more than 100,000 lives a year.

Generally, herbs have been found to provide additional nutrients that restore health, protect the immune system, normalize body functions, and impart natural relief from health-harming emotions. Thus, herbal therapy is an effective, natural way to help the body heal itself.

In the United States today, many herbs—including kava—are approved dietary supplements. As defined by the United States government, a dietary supplement is a vitamin, mineral, herb or other botanical, an amino acid, and any dietary substance used to supplement the diet. The term also includes concentrates, metabolites, extracts, or combinations of herbs and botanical ingredients.

Under the Dietary Supplement Health and Education Act of 1994, supplement manufacturers can't say that products diagnose, treat, prevent, or cure disease. If they do, the product must be regarded as a drug and then must meet the safety and effectiveness standards for drugs. So if a kava-supplement manufacturer were to advertise that its kava product cures stress or anxiety, the company would find itself on the regulatory hot seat with the FDA. However, manufacturers may make nutrition support statements about their products—statements that describe how the product functions in the body. Thus, it's perfectly legal for a manufacturer to promote kava's ability to aid in relaxation. Also, supplement labels must carry the following disclaimer: "This statement has not been evaluated by the Food and Drug Administration. This product is not intended to diagnose, treat, cure, or prevent any disease."

The term "kava" is the name of the plant as well as the beverage made from it. In some books and articles you may find kava described as a drug, an intoxicant, or a narcotic, although it is a legal, approved supplement. The reason kava is given these other descriptions is most likely due to the intoxicating effect more potent forms of kava—specifically the freshly ground root served in the

South Pacific—has on the body. Raw root is unavailable in the United States or Europe. Instead, products are made from processed, dry root powder, which is much weaker, so it's quite unlikely that you would obtain the kava "high" experienced by South Pacific islanders.

THE GIFT OF TRANQUILLITY FROM THE PACIFIC

Today kava is found in three distinct cultural regions of the world collectively referred to as Oceania: Melanesia, which includes the island countries of Fiji, Vanuatu (formerly New Hebrides), New Guinea, and Papua New Guinea; Polynesia, which includes Hawaii, Tahiti, the Marquesas Islands, Wallis, Futuna, Western and American Samoa, and Tonga; and Micronesia, which includes Pohnpei and Australia. These areas are scattered over nearly a third of the earth's surface and include some ten thousand islands. As then president George Bush told a summit of Pacific island leaders in 1990: "Like a string of pearls spread out across the sea, each nation is unique, each is precious, and each has something to contribute to the value of the whole."

One of Oceania's many contributions is, of course, kava—a true gift of tranquillity. Kava is woven into the very fabric of Oceanian life—religiously, socially, and politically—and is thought to be one of the reasons behind the islanders' laid-back way of life. Kava, with its ritual procedure for preparation and use, is one custom that is common to all peoples of Oceania. Consequently, it has attracted a great deal of attention from anthropologists, botanists, chemists, pharmacologists, doctors, and even archaeologists.

Kava is best understood when it is recognized that every culture in the world has some type of special plant customarily used to induce mind-altering and mood-altering effects. Betel nut, one of the world's most popular plants, is chewed, mashed, or pulverized by the peoples of India, Malaysia, and Polynesia and used as a stimulant. In southeast Mexico, Oaxacan tribes consume the psilocybe mushroom for its hallucinogenic and muscle-relaxing effects. African pygmies smoke their psychoactive cannabis, derived from the hemp plant, and Andean natives chew their coca leaf, the source of the illegal drug cocaine. From 1891 until about 1908, the Coca-Cola Company formulated its popular cola drink with cocaine from coca leaves and caffeine from kola nuts, a plant whose seeds are high in the stimulant caffeine. Today Coke's products are made with caffeine and natural flavorings.

More familiarly, tobacco leaves contain a powerfully addictive substance known as nicotine. From the beans of the coffee tree and the leaves of the tea bush come caffeine, the most widely used drug in the world. Thus, a huge array of various plants yields various natural chemicals, ranging from the benign to the very dangerous. In moderate doses, kava is on the benign end of the spectrum.

WHY KAVA WORKS

For centuries kava has been used as a folk medicine to treat a vast number of ailments. These have included headaches, joint pain, bladder problems, gonorrhea, stomach problems, leprosy, skin diseases, weight loss, sleeping problems, and tuberculosis.

Since the 1800s much research has been devoted to identifying why kava provides such amazing therapeutic benefits. In fact, kava is one of the most extensively studied herbs, with hundreds of scientific studies backing up its healing properties and verifying its power as a therapeutic agent capable of conferring remarkable benefits. For example, kava:

- relieves everyday stress
- significantly lowers anxiety after only one week of use
- effectively manages long-term anxiety
- is as effective as some prescription drugs in reducing serious anxiety
- induces relaxation
- acts as a muscle relaxant
- has analgesic (pain-relieving) properties
- may help prevent abnormal blood clotting
- acts as an anticonvulsive
- may protect the brain
- may help smokers and alcoholics kick the habit
- improves alertness, memory, and reaction time
- significantly reduces menopausal symptoms (anxiety and depression)

Kava's therapeutic effects are due to at least fifteen different lipidlike compounds, collectively known by two interchangeable names, either "kavapyrones" or "kavalactones." Most of these compounds produce physical and mental relaxation without causing addiction or harmful side effects when the herb is taken in moderate doses.

There are many varieties of kava plants, and their concentrations of kavalactones vary. Certain types of kava may be richer in kavalactones that impart the feeling of calm most kava-users enjoy, while other varieties may be filled with kavalactones that produce nausea and headaches.

Kava is a relatively new herb to the United States, but not to Germany, where it has been available by prescription since 1920. Approximately 350,000 prescriptions for kava are written annually in Germany for anxiety-related disorders. In 1990 kava was approved by the German Commission E, Germany's equivalent to our FDA, for treating anxiety, stress, and restlessness. French pharmaceutical companies also import a great deal of kava for medicinal use.

The most significant body of research on herbs—including kava—and their clinical applications comes from the observations made during the thousands of years in which they have been used in Europe. And the best clinical reference tool is the German Commission E monograph, a publication describing scores of herbs and their therapeutic applications.

To date, very few clinical trials have been conducted in America; most kava studies have been done in Europe. However, the National Institute of Mental Health in the United States is considering a closer look at kava.

In the United States kava is available without a doctor's prescription. It comes in several forms: capsules, standardized extracts, dried ground root, teas, and multiherb formulations. Taken as directed in moderate dosages, these forms of kava are quite gentle, and certainly not as strong as the kind used by South Pacific islanders, who grind fresh kava root daily and brew a quite potent, mind-altering beverage.

IS KAVA SAFE?

Kava has a long history of safe usage. Modern pharmaceutical grades of kava extracts, standardized for kavalactone strength and quality, have passed the extensive safety scrutiny required for drug registration in Germany.

To promote kava's safety and avoid any regulatory problems connected with its use, twenty-one manufacturers of herbal supplements banded together in 1996 to form the Kava General Committee. Its thrust has been to play up kava's therapeutic value. One of the group's first actions was to commission a safety review of the herb by the Herb Research Foundation of Boulder, Colorado, and under the auspices of the American Botanical Council, a trade association of herbal supplement manufacturers. This safety review, which included information from several well-designed, well-controlled German studies, helped catapult kava into the limelight as a superior therapeutic remedy.

In the kava review, more than eighty sources of information were consulted to search out facts about the herb's chemical, therapeutic, and cultural properties. In its report, the Herb Research Foundation concluded that kava is virtually a safe and effective anti-anxiety agent and muscle relaxant when taken in normal therapeutic doses.

Further, the German Commission E monograph on kava states that there are no side effects, except with extended, continual intake. And those side effects include temporary yellowing of the skin, hair, and nails. Kava is not without other side effects, too, particularly with irresponsible use. Megadoses, for example, can cause muscular weakness, visual problems, dizziness, and drying of the skin. Long-term use can lead to high blood pressure, protein metabolism problems, blood cell abnormalities, or liver damage. Among South Pacific islanders, continual chewing of the root destroys the tooth enamel.

But when taken for short-term usage in recommended doses for stress, anxiety, and other mood disorders, kava is one of the safest agents available—certainly far safer than many prescription medications.

There have been no studies to date on whether kava causes cancer, produces fetal malformations, or causes genetic mutations. However, kava use by islanders for centuries gives no indication of any of these effects.

As attention on this once-obscure herb intensifies, more and more consumers are flocking to health food stores, pharmacies, and Wal-Marts everywhere to check out this amazing supplement for themselves. What we now know about it, from its fascinating history to its present-day medicinal value, forms a persuasive body of knowledge that kava is truly nature's solution to stress, anxiety, and many other ills. Just read on, and you'll find out why.

CHAPTER 2

Kava Lore

Kava has been used for more than three thousand years in the South Pacific, in various rites and customs as well as for medicinal purposes. The plant has long been an important part of various ceremonies, and these include welcoming distinguished visitors, marking the beginning and end of work, preparing for journeys and ocean voyages, proclaiming laws and codes of conduct, reconciling with enemies, and blessing kings and chiefs. Kava has been used informally as well. Elder men in villages had a cup first thing in the morning, while older family members enjoyed a cup before dinner.

But in most Oceanian places where kava is consumed, its major significance has traditionally been religious. And with this religious tradition comes a wealth of fascinating history and lore.

KAVA AND RELIGION

Long ago, and to a limited extent today, islanders worshiped a bevy of gods, as did the ancient Greeks and

Romans. The three major gods, known by various names throughout Oceania, were Tangaloa, or Tagaloa, the ruler of the sky, who was often credited with the creation of the earth; Hikule'o, ruler of the underworld; and Maui, a hero demigod who could change his form, do magic, and tame the forces of nature. Maui has been nicknamed the "Polynesian Hercules." In South Pacific mythology, there were also gods of fire, storms, and wind, among others, as well as various supernatural beings such as spirits, fairies, elves, and demons.

Ancestor worship has long been a part of island religion, too. Via oral histories passed down through generations, many Pacific people know the stories of their founding ancestors, who migrated to the islands and ultimately were revered as gods. Their faces or bodies are carved in wood, stone, or ivory and occupy treasured places in people's homes. And even more recently departed ancestors are worshiped. The personal possessions of a dead relative are often kept as objects of worship.

Since ancient times, kava has been interwoven into South Pacific religious worship, usually presented as an offering to the gods. In Samoa, for example, it was traditional for the head of the household to pour kava on the ground before dinner was eaten, as part of the blessing. And in formal ceremonies, the priest always offered the first cup to the gods. In Tonga, people left a small piece of the kava root beside a consecrated house or grave as worship to the gods or in memory of the departed soul of a loved one or tribal chief. On some Tongan islands, natives threw shavings of kava root into the sea while praying to the shark god, Sekatoa. The Tannese on Vanuatu spit out kava in honor of the gods, and then made short prayers to their ancestors. In Hawaii, the kahuna (a type of priest) believed kava was the offering most favored by the gods.

For many South Pacific peoples, kava drinking has also been a way of accessing the spirit world so as to commune with the gods and ancestors. After consuming kava, people prayed to their ancestors, or just conversed with them about daily events, to obtain some sort of revelation. Similarly, priests drank kava to induce a trancelike state that they believed facilitated communication with the supernatural. Trances were thought to be the vehicle through which gods and ancestors could inhabit the body of the priest, a type of divine channeling induced by kava.

People also drank the herbal brew to receive messages from their ancestors, believing that kava made it easier for the dead to commune with the living. Tranquilized by kava, they would sit and wait for inspirational messages and knowledge from their departed forebears. It was not uncommon for the living to believe they could commune with the dead through their dreams. Kava makes dreams very vivid; thus, people used it to intensify dreams and promote better contact with ancestral spirits.

But kava is also connected to sorcery, usually to making magic more effective. Vanuatu magicians, for example, spit out kava to subdue unruly women. In Fiji, a person who wanted someone dead recruited a sorcerer who would first prepare the kava and then pour it on the grave of an ancestor of the intended victim. If the victim died, the ritual was repeated. And in some Pacific regions, people drank kava mixed with a dead person's bodily fluids to divine the identity of the sorcerer who had caused the death.

In the mid to late 1800s and the early 1900s, Protestant and Catholic missionaries began setting up missions on Pacific islands. Generally, their attitude toward kava drinking was one of disapproval. They labeled the beverage the "devil's drink" and fought kava, along with its associated religious practices, as best they could. This was very hard to do, because kava was so enmeshed in the rituals, customs, and social order of native societies. However, they were successful in eradicating kava from several parts of the Pacific, including Hawaii and Tahiti.

When Presbyterian missionaries first arrived on the island of Tanna in Vanuatu in 1854, they tolerated kava somewhat. By the 1870s and 1880s, converts were required to abstain from kava drinking in order to take holy communion. Other than this restriction, there were no moves to obliterate its use among the islanders. Some missionaries wanted to fire any mission teacher who drank kava, but this was largely met with opposition.

Many Tannese converts felt that Christianity and kava drinking were compatible, and so they continued to enjoy the native brew. However, other converts were even more vehemently opposed to kava drinking than the missionaries. They fiercely attacked kava and the customs attached to it. For example, converts and missionaries were successful in enacting a law (known as the Tanna Law) that forbade people from drinking kava, transporting it along the roads, and using it in ceremonies. Kava drinkers were frequently arrested, even though they were just practicing their native customs.

The Tanna law was revoked in 1912 after islanders pled their case to British officials (Vanuatu was then a formal colony under joint British and French rule). However, damage to the structure of pagan society had already been done, and many native customs were in shambles. By 1939 Christians outnumbered pagans two to one. The missionaries forbade dancing, ancestor worship, the practice of magic—and the ritual consumption of kava.

At some point during this period, a mysterious man named John Frum appeared. Little is known about him except that he may have been a trader and that he showed up frequently at prohibited kava-drinking sessions on the island. Frum told people to hold on to their customs, to stop attending mission churches, and to drink kava openly. His message spread, and there was an increase in kava drinking. It was, in fact, excessive—an act of rebellion against what was seen as the oppressive influence of the church.

An entire cult has grown up around John Frum—a cult that is today upheld by a few thousand of Tanna's twenty-two thousand residents. His followers see Frum as a messiah who speaks all languages and travels to and from America through one of the volcanoes on Tanna. Adherents to the cult eagerly await Frum's return and with it his promise that they will share the white man's wealth—trucks, refrigerators, factories, and other material items. On Tanna there is a John Frum church, John Frum disciples, a John Frum sabbath (Friday nights), and a John Frum Day (February 15).

The John Frum movement on Tanna is part of a phenomenon known as the "cargo cult," an odd type of religious sect that develops when modern conveniences such as radios or electricity are introduced into cultures that have never seen them before. Cargo cultists believe that these goods belong to them, and that with the help of ancestral spirits, they can acquire them. Prophets in these cults preach that the arrival of cargo (foreign goods) will usher in a period of prosperity.

Another active cargo cult on Vanuatu is the Prince Philip Movement. Some islanders think Britain's Prince Philip is a personification of an ancestral spirit, and they often display his photo as an act of adoration.

Cults aside, with the passage of time many missionaries relaxed their restrictions on kava, and in many places today, kava is incorporated into worship services. Even so, some scholars believe that the strong missionary influence in the nineteenth century was responsible for eradicating kava drinking from some islands altogether.

Since 1900, Christian denominations have been the majority in the South Pacific, with Catholics in the lead, Protestants next, and Anglicans third. Evangelical and Pentecostal Christians have all been gaining converts, too. By the year 2000, roughly 83 percent of the population in the South Pacific will be Christian, according to the Global Evangelization Movement. Other religions in the region include Buddhists, Hindus, and Muslims. Those who still practice native religions comprise about one percent of the population.

WHERE DID KAVA COME FROM?

Botanically known as *Piper methysticum,* kava is a member of the *Piper* genus, a broad biological class that comprises about 2,000 species of plants. Kava thus has many relatives in its genus. One is betel *(Piper betle L.),* whose leaves are chewed in various parts of Asia and the South Pacific to produce a stimulant effect. Another is kavakava 'ulie *(Macropiper puberulum),* native to Fiji and Tonga. Its leaves are valued for their healing properties. The plant is not used as a beverage but is, rather, made into an infusion for treating skin inflammations and stomachaches. In South America, two of the Piper species, *Piper interitum* and *Piper cryptodon,* are used as tobacco substitutes by the Amazon Indians. The black pepper on your dinner table is *Piper nigrum.* A number of other Piper species are prized as culinary spices or medicinal drugs in various parts of the world.

The kava cultivated in the South Pacific is most probably a descendant of a plant called "wild kava" or *Piper wichmannii.* All kava is believed to have originated on the volcanically formed islands of Vanuatu, where the most potent form is grown today, although some botanists believe it was once native to New Guinea and to the Solomon Islands.

According to noted kava researcher and geneticist Vincent Lebot in his book, *Kava: The Pacific Elixir,* Vanuatu islanders were probably the first to discover the psychoactive properties of *Piper wichmannii.* After concocting and sampling a particularly good batch of kava, they selected the *Piper wichmannii* plants that produced it, cut off its stems, and planted them. Over time, this "cloning" process led to the development of the domesticated varieties that are today cultivated in the South Pacific.

It was customary for seafaring islanders who migrated to new lands to take their indigenous plants with them on their voyages. After all, they didn't know if the land awaiting them would be endowed with the plants to which they were accustomed. Thus, from Vanuatu, kava was probably carried by canoe to Fiji, where it is called *yagona* (from an Oceanian word meaning "bitter"). Fijians most likely took it with them to Polynesia, and the people there dubbed it *kawa,* which also means "bitter."

ORIGIN MYTHS

Although no one knows for sure the exact origin of the plant, Pacific people have their own fascinating myths about how kava came into being—myths that reveal the almost mystical and sacred position kava holds in their cultures. These myths tell of kava's great value and divine bestowal, signifying the reverence islanders attach to kava today.

According to Lebot, nearly all kava origin myths fall into two classifications: tales in which a god comes down from the heavens to give the gift of kava to the people, or stories of how and where the plant first began to grow.

Samoan legend, for example, has it that a beautiful girl named Ui was sacrificed to the Sun god as part of the annual sun ceremony. He was so enamored of her that he took her for his wife. Ui became pregnant and was allowed to return to earth to give birth. But during her descent to earth, she miscarried. The fetus floated on the water and was cared for by a hermit crab. Named Tagaloa Ui, the child grew up and taught mortals how to make a special drink called kava kava and how to use it with reverence in religious ceremonies.

The story goes on to say that the very first kava ceremony was conducted by a man named Pava, whose son mocked the way he prepared the root for drinking. This attitude angered Tagaloa Ui, and using a coconut frond as a knife, he cut Pava's son in half. Tagaloa Ui said to Pava: "This is the food for the kava. This is your part and this mine." But deeply grieved, Pava could not eat his own son. He prepared a second round of kava made from Tagaloa's own grove and offered it to the god. In an act of mercy, Tagaloa did not drink it but poured it over his half of the dead son. The two parts of the body came together, and Pava's son was brought back to life.

Another Samoan legend has it that kava was the drink of the gods, originally found only in heaven. The god Tagaloa descended from heaven one day with two assistants to go fishing. The assistants caught some fish and presented them to Tagaloa, who wanted some kava to drink with them. Because there was none on earth, the god sent his assistants back to heaven to get a kava root. They pulled up an entire plant, however, and Tagaloa scattered its parts all over the earth, where it thrived. A downpour of rain provided the water to infuse the kava root. Thus, the drink of the gods was introduced to people on earth.

Sometimes a hero, rather than a god, bestows the gift of kava. In southeastern Irian Jaya, the story is told of a hero named Wonati who could change at will into a stork. In that form, he flew to a river and then morphed back into a man who began chewing kava, a plant that was unfamiliar to the people. After teaching them how to use it, Wonati changed back into a stork and flew away. He became a man again and got married. The first thing he did was teach his father-in-law how to plant and cultivate a kava garden. For the cuttings, Wonati plucked the hairs from his armpits.

In a Vanuatu legend recorded and told by Lebot in his book, a young woman refused to marry a certain stranger. A struggle ensued between her brother and the rejected suitor, who accidentally let loose an arrow that struck and killed the woman. Full of sorrow, the brother buried his sister. After a week, an unusual plant sprouted over her tomb, and the brother decided to let it grow. A year later, the brother, who often visited his sister's grave site, saw a rat eat the plant's roots and die. (Rats do, in fact, chew kava.) Still mourning over his sister's death, he wanted to die and so he ate the roots in an effort to end his own life. But his suicide attempt failed. What happened next was quite miraculous: All sorrow and unhappiness left him. Afterward, he returned often to the grave to eat the magic root, and he introduced it to others.

In many Tongan and Fijian myths, kava is said to sprout from the body of lepers. Such tales probably developed from the fact that prolonged overconsumption of kava can create a scaly skin condition that resembles leprosy. And in other island myths, the plant springs from kangaroos, corpses, the vagina or breasts of a dead woman, or from the body of a female deity.

Further, Polynesian myth is filled with tales of a dreaded demon named Miru who lived in Avaiki, the netherworld. Miru's favorite meal was the spirit of a dead person. To prepare the spirit food, Miru would first intoxicate her victims with kava (called "Miru's own"), cook them in her ever-burning oven, and later devour their spirits.

FROM VANUATU TO TONGA

Among the most fascinating myths surrounding kava is one that recounts how the plant and beverage made their way from Vanuatu, its probable country of origin, to neighboring Tonga. This myth is rooted in and intertwined with some fascinating historical facts.

Writing in *The Journal of Polynesian Society,* scholar David Luders notes that historically there was once a thriving trade between the two countries—until the mid–fifteenth century, circa 1447, five years before the volcanic explosion of the island of Kuwae sometime in 1452. (Kuwae was formerly a part of what is today central Vanuatu.) This volcanic eruption was of cataclysmic proportions—considered by geologists one of the eight most destructive eruptions in the past ten thousand years. The island shattered into pieces, and 30 million cubic meters of rock and magma were hurled into the air. Dust encircled the earth and hung in the atmosphere for at least three years, according to geological records, partially blotting out the sun and creating a minor ice age. Global devastation followed, with crop damage and famines from Mexico to China.

This true-life natural disaster spawned an intriguing kava myth. In island mythology, there was a female deity named Pufafine, who was synonymous with the land—a type of earth goddess. Kava grew from her body (the land of Kuwae). The islanders farmed the land, and the chiefs used kava to communicate with their ancestors and spirits.

Myth and history then converge. Historically, it is known that at some point in the early fifteenth century, Tongans began journeying to Vanuatu, where they discovered kava. At first, they began taking home the leaves and stems of wild kava. This form of kava is thought to have been much stronger than the domesticated variety and to have contained kavalactones that imparted some nasty side effects such as nausea and headaches. Eventually the Tongans learned of the existence of a better, more highly prized kava, which grew on the island of Kuwae—a kava that was fiercely guarded because it was used by the chiefs only. In fact the Kuwae chiefs kept the kava plantations secret from the Tongans. Nonetheless, the Tongans discovered the good kava and ultimately plundered the plantations, leaving very little.

Back to the mythical portion of the story: The Tongans' greed so infuriated Pufafine that she became pregnant—but pregnant with a vengeance. She gave birth—a birth that symbolically represents the actual volcanic eruption on the island of Kuwae. In the myth the ocean and skies turn red—which actually would have occurred following an explosion of this magnitude. Thus, the myth is an attempt to explain the cause of a real volcano—yet it is a record of history, albeit a history cloaked in mythic symbols.

KAVA TALES

Kava is a supporting character in scores of myths and legends in which gods, heroes, and villains take part in preparing and drinking the powerful potion. In one legend, kava even has a role to play in the origin of coconuts, probably the best known of all South Pacific crops.

As the story goes, a mother was drawing saltwater from the sea for cooking purposes and accidentally caught an eel. She took it home and gave it to her daughter Sina as a plaything. After finding Sina in tears one day, her parents assumed the eel had bitten the child and decided the creature was the incarnation of an evil god. The family fled their home to escape the eel. But the eel chased after them.

The family came to a village and was welcomed by a chief, who invited them in for something to drink. Sina accepted the invitation on the condition that the chief get rid of the eel. So the chief prepared a batch of kava and mixed it with some poisonous plants from the jungle. The first cup was offered to the eel, who gulped it down and began to die. The eel's last words to Sina were that they part in peace. He instructed her to cook his dead body, but afterward plant his head in the ground. Sina followed his instructions, and the head grew into a coconut tree.

JUDEO-CHRISTIAN/PAGAN LEGENDS

Beginning in the 1800s, when Christian missionaries first began to evangelize to South Pacific peoples, "newer myths" were created around kava, and pagan beliefs became fused with Judeo-Christian beliefs. In his book *The Abandoned Narcotic,* Ron Brunton recounts the following: A myth existed in Tanna, the largest island of Vanuatu, that at one time the entire world was Tanna. (The word *Tanna* actually means "earth.") Then Jesus made Adam and Eve, who broke His commandments by eating food before they had been told which foods were allowed and which were prohibited. Once Jesus discovered that the couple had already eaten, He decided to withhold from them certain knowledge and power.

The myth—obviously an aberration of biblical accounts—continues on episodically to conclude with Moses, who received power and knowledge from Jesus in the form of a stone tablet. Moses instructed the people (the Tannese) to think and act like him. But they disobeyed. One man made an image of a bull, and the people begin to worship it—an account similar to the story of the golden calf found in the Book of Exodus in the Bible. This act of idol worship infuriated Moses, who dropped the stone tablet, breaking it into ten pieces. At the same time, Tanna broke apart to become all the lands of the world. The European people, who had been faithful to Moses' instructions, left for the newly created parts of the world, taking all power and knowledge with them. Moses' son felt sorry for the Tannese and so gave them foods, magic—and kava, which became their source of power.

TRUE STORIES: KAVA "DISCOVERED" BY WESTERNERS

So much for myth and legend! The historical accounts of kava's "discovery" by Europeans are just as fascinating. The first Westerners ever to observe and record the preparation and ritual consumption of kava were Jacob LeMaire and William Schouten, two Dutch explorers voyaging through the Pacific as early as 1616. Its use was well entrenched in island communities when Captain James Cook made his historic voyages through the South Pacific. During his first voyage (1768–71), it was the responsibility of Swedish botanist Daniel Solander and artist Sydney Parkinson to make sketches of the newly discovered plant. This task was essential in the age before photography. Parkinson ultimately produced more than twelve hundred drawings of various animals and plants— the most detailed pictorial record of any eighteenth-century voyage.

Cook himself was probably the first explorer to ever try kava, although he didn't like it much. He recorded the following entry in his journal in October 1773 upon visiting the island of Tonga for the first time: ". . . those people who came first off to us in the Canoes brought with them some [of the pepper plant] Root of which they made their drink which they sent aboard before they came in themselves. One would not wish for a better sign of friendship than this; can we make a friend more welcome than by setting before him the best liquor in our possession or than can be got? In this manner did those friendly people receive us; I never visited the old Chief but he ordered some of the root just mentioned to be brought me and would also set some of his people to chew it and prepared the liquor, notwithstanding I seldom tasted any . . ."

A naturalist who had sailed with him, Johann Georg Forster, officially named kava *Piper methysticum* in 1777. Translated, this means "intoxicating pepper," reflecting its kinship to the pepper family and its physical effect on the body (*methys* is the Greek work for "drunken").

In a bygone era, the drink was prepared by virgin boys (and sometimes girls) who chewed a wad of the fresh root until its fibers were thoroughly broken down. Chewing supposedly released more of the plant's active ingredients due to the action of enzymes in the saliva that break down kava's pulp. Chewers had to have strong teeth and jaws, clean mouths, and be free from any disease. They rinsed their mouths out with clean water prior to chew-

ing and were not supposed to wet the root with saliva as
they chewed. Observers of this method of preparation
have said it is amazing that very little saliva was actually
mixed in with the chewed root.

In most Pacific places, chewing kava was specifically a
male task. Archaeologists who study the skeletal remains
of prehistoric Oceanian peoples theorize that kava chewing was responsible for the high incidence of temporo-
mandibular joint (TMJ) degeneration among men. TMJ
problems occur when the cartilage and bone of the jaw
break down, usually due to overuse. The discovery of
TMJ degeneration among primitive men also proves that
kava use has been in existence since prehistoric times,
perhaps as early as 1100 B.C.

The masticated, partially digested kava was spit onto a
banana leaf or directly into a kava bowl. Water was
poured over the mass, which was soaked until the concoc-
tion reached its desired strength. The pulp was strained
out through the strands of the bark of a native tree or part
of a coconut palm and poured into coconut shells for
consumption during rituals. For hygienic reasons, this
traditional method of kava preparation has been largely
abandoned in most islands. (In Tanna on Vanuatu, kava is
still masticated as part of its preparation.)

In 1773 Forster had an opportunity to observe two
Polynesians prepare and drink kava in Captain Cook's
cabin. Forster described the scene in his book *A Voyage
Round the World in His Britannic Majesty's Sloop,* published
in 1777:

"[Kava] is made in the most disgustful manner than
can be imagined, from the juice contained in the roots of
a species of pepper-tree. This root is cut small and the
pieces chewed by several people, who spit the masticated
mass into a bowl, where some water (milk) of coconuts is

poured upon it. They then strain it through the fibres of coconuts, squeezing the chips, till all their juices mix with the coconut milk; and the whole liquor is decanted into another bowl. They swallow this nauseous stuff as fast as possible; and some old topers value themselves on being able to empty a great number of bowls."

Forster was also the first to document the effect that overconsumption of kava by native islanders had on the skin by writing that "the skin dries up and exfoliates in little scales." Today, this skin disease is known as kava dermopathy.

Captain James King, who took up the official journal writing after Cook's death at the hands of Hawaiians in 1779, was among the earliest explorers to describe and record an actual kava ceremony, which took place in Hawaii in January 1779. He wrote: ". . . the natives sat down fronting us, and began to cut up the baked hog, to peel the vegetables, and break the cocoa-nuts; whilst others employed themselves in brewing the ava [kava]; which is done by chewing it, in the same manner as the Friendly Islands. . . . The ava was then handed round and after we had tasted it Koah and Pareea began to pull the flesh of the hog in pieces, and to put it into our mouths."

In the South Pacific today, the stories and myths surrounding this fascinating plant are kept alive, passed down from generation to generation, and often retold whenever islanders gather to enjoy their kava.

CHAPTER 3

Kava, Kava, Everywhere

Just as the British have their teatime and the Americans their cocktail hour, islanders in the South Pacific have their own special time to drink kava, usually around sunset after work and before supper. This tradition probably originates from old legends saying that the spirits are present only after sunset.

The revered place kava holds in island culture has not changed much with the passage of time. According to one Polynesian: "It is important to us in many ways—socially, culturally, and religiously. Kava helps everyone feel part of the community and the village."

KAVA CULTIVATION

Kava is a slow-growing perennial shrub usually cultivated on patches of swampy land, plantations, hillsides, or in moist forests. To thrive, it requires a tropical climate with much rainfall and fertile, well-drained soil. The plant is an attractive shrub, distinguished by its lovely, heart-shaped leaves and woody, jointed stems. In some places, it can grow as high as twenty feet, although commercial kava plants are usually harvested at seven or eight feet. Kava is not a seasonal crop, but grows year round.

The parts of the plant cultivated for its active ingredients are the root, or stump, and the ruffle of lateral roots growing from it. The roots contain a yellow-colored resin that is rich in kavalactones. An entire root system can weigh as much as one hundred pounds, and a dried root weighs just 20 percent of its fresh weight.

The plant has male and female flowers, but is sterile. No fruits or seeds have ever been seen on kava plants. Thus, kava must be planted much like sugarcane—by sticking sections of the stalk into the ground or well-watered beds and sheltering them from direct sunlight and wind. The plant depends entirely on humans for its perpetuation. Many botanists feel that this method of propagation has made kava populations less healthy and more disease prone. It is not unusual to see losses of up to 60 percent of a crop yield.

Kava is often grown under the protection of shade-providing crops such as banana, coconut, mango, or papaya trees. Kava growers still test the strength and potency of their own plants by drinking kava made from the rootstock. If the kava is weak, the grower will not clone, or replant, its stem cuttings.

The plants are considered mature at seven years old, although kava grown as a commercial crop is often harvested at two to three years old. The older the root, however, the stronger is its strength and flavor. Kava plants are quite different from region to region, varying widely in odor, flavor, and potency. Some varieties are reserved only for certain ceremonies, some for medicinal purposes, and still others for everyday consumption. Each variety has a different name, too, often derived from its color; the characteristics of its stems, leaves, or roots; legendary origins; or the name of the first grower to have cultivated the clone. Natives are very familiar with the qualities of each variety. In his book *Kava: Medicine Hunting in Paradise,* author Chris Kilham recounts how one islander pointed out a yellow-stalked kava grown on Vanuatu that is so strong it makes the drinker sleep for two days.

On Fiji, there are five varieties, three white and two black. The white kava is supposed to be the best, but it takes longer to grow—at least four years. Black kava, on the other hand, can be harvested in two to three years and is thus cultivated for commercial use.

Distributors who sell the root worldwide typically have to negotiate with village chiefs to purchase the roots. More commonly, kava growers sell their crop directly to traders, or middlemen.

In many South Seas villages, kava is harvested directly from the jungle, or straight from someone's own crop. The men dig up fresh roots, but replant a few stalks of good crop to perpetuate the supply, and immediately begin to ready them for drinking. (In other places, namely Fiji, Samoa, and Tonga, the root is usually dried first.) The roots are cleaned, scraped, and cut into small pieces. On the island of Tanna in Vanuatu, this work is generally a social time when men, young and old, discuss matters of the day. The root is then pulverized by one of several methods, depending on the country and its customs, and strained to produce the beverage.

Freshly harvested kava is quite perishable and must be protected from mold and rotting. Stumps and roots are washed thoroughly, then usually sliced and dried in the sun, or by a hot-air dryer to remove most of the moisture. After drying, the material may be placed in jute sacks, or ground into a powder. Chunks of the stump and root are also shipped in bulk to European pharmaceutical companies for further processing into extracts.

KAVA COUNTRIES

Kava is truly a Pacific potion—the official drink of the South Seas. Although it grows throughout the South Pacific, certain regions are more strongly associated with it than others. These are described below.

FIJI

The Fiji Islands, once infamously known as the Cannibal Islands, form a horseshoe-shaped chain of 322 islands (100 of them inhabited) and are among the most popular travel destinations in the South Pacific. Volcanically formed, Fiji was discovered in 1643 by Abel Tasman, a mariner who first sighted the island but never really set foot on it. The first seaman to describe Fiji to Europeans was Captain William Bligh of *Bounty* fame in the late 1700s.

Independent since 1970, Fiji is today a lush tropical playground with posh hotels, a wide range of recreational activities, water sports, nightlife, and historic sites. The Fijians have done a wonderful job of preserving their many island traditions and customs, including kava drinking. Nearly 40,000 people are employed in the kava industry in Fiji. In a bygone era, kava was reserved for tribal chiefs only, but today kava is the national drink of Fiji. Tourists are often invited to drink kava on social occasions. Turning down the invitation is considered an insult in Fijian society.

Botanists categorize kava in sophisticated ways, for instance, as "chemotypes," (based on the chemical makeup of the plant); as "morphotypes," (based on the physical characteristics); and as "zymotypes," (based on the genetic markers used to determine whether one type of plant evolved from another). But South Sea islanders use a more garden-variety approach for categorizing their kava, usually based on its strength. For example, Fijian kava farmers "grade" their kava according to the concentration of kavalactones in the various parts of the plant. The highest concentration is obtained from the plant's lateral roots—a kava known as *waka* grade. Other grades are *lewena* and *kasa,* both harvested from the base of the plant's stems. These forms of kava are less concentrated with kavalactones and therefore less costly than *waka* grade (the most expensive of the three). Fiji is the only South Pacific country that classifies its kava in this manner.

Fijian kava is not as strong as that which grows on Vanuatu. One reason may be that Fijian farmers harvest young kava plants. (On Vanuatu, the supply of older— and thus stronger—kava is so plentiful that growers can afford to harvest as much as they need.)

Kava is an important medicine on Fiji. In fact, Fijian spiritual leaders are called *dauvagunu,* which, translated literally, means an "expert at drinking kava." A dauvagunu uses kava to access a spirit force named *Vu* in order to help cure a patient. Fiji's spiritual healers also believe they can see into the future and divine herbal remedies after drinking kava.

VANUATU

Although Vanuatu is believed to have been populated since before 3000 B.C., it was "discovered" in 1606 by a Spanish explorer, Pedro Fernandez de Quirós. Vanuatu is a Y-shaped string of eighty-two islands originally formed by volcanoes and layered with limestone plateaus. *Vanuatu,* which means "land eternal," is tropical and largely unspoiled, with thick rainforests and sparkling beaches. Interestingly, the country welcomes more cruise-ship visitors than any other South Pacific island. The tiny nation gained its independence from joint British-French rule on July 30, 1980.

The kava consumed in Vanuatu is the strongest anywhere in the South Pacific, with the islands of Tanna and Pentecost especially noted for their potent brews. Adding to its potency is the fact that it is prepared from the raw, fresh roots, whereas in Fiji and elsewhere it is made from dried rootstock. Kava is grown commercially on Vanuatu and has become an important cash crop for the islanders. There are more varieties of kava growing on Vanuatu than anywhere else in the South Pacific. Kava drinking on Vanuatu is more social than ceremonial. The plant is widely used to treat physical illnesses, as well.

Up until about twenty years ago, however, kava drinking was discouraged by missionaries and government officials. But today this opposition has largely faded, and kava has become an important cultural symbol. Kava drinking has come to represent *kastom,* the political traditions that perpetuate the country's national unity and identity. Political ceremonies, from the opening of Parliament to the celebration of independence day, often include kava drinking.

In Vanuatu kava is usually ground using a mortar and pestle. The mortars may be large pipes, hollowed-out wood, or even old World War II shell casings. However, chewing the root is still practiced in some parts of Vanuatu, particularly on Tanna. Tannese youths who have been circumcised (a symbol that they are full-fledged members of the male community) masticate the root for older men. Adults may chew kava for a friend or guest, as an honor.

If a man chews his own kava, it is a sign that he is upset with the others.

The Tannese men chew the kava until it reaches an appropriate consistency, then spit it out onto coconut or banana leaves. Each drinker receives a separate fist-sized wad of masticated kava. Young boys are dispensed to bring fresh water, which is poured over the kava. A circumcised virgin boy mixes the kava with water and strains it through a coconut frond into a coconut-shell bowl. The "leftover" kava pulp is set aside to be used for a second, weaker round.

Silently the drinker downs the entire bowl at once, then spits on the ground—an act called the *tamafa*, which is a prayer to his ancestor. As is customary, the drinker then touches the empty bowl to the ground before passing it to the next man. If he passes the bowl without touching it to the ground, superstition has it that all the power of the kava will go to the next drinker.

Vanuatu is one of the South Sea countries that has a brisk "nakamal" business. A nakamal is a kava bar, where locals and tourists alike can enjoy a quaff or two of freshly ground and strained kava. In 1980 the country had just a few nakamals; today it has more than sixty scattered throughout the towns and villages. The Vanuatu government frowns upon alcohol consumption, but favors kava use. The reason: Kava imparts a tranquil sociability, whereas alcohol—a depressant—can lead to bad behavior and violence.

HAWAII

Called *awa* or *ava* in Hawaii, kava was first brought to the Hawaiian islands by Polynesian settlers. In 1779 Captain James Cook and crew observed that nowhere in the South Pacific was kava drunk more copiously than in

Hawaii. In fact, they felt that Hawaiians were quite addicted to the brew. For roughly a fourteen-year period in the 1800s, there was a thriving kava industry in Hawaii, and much kava was exported. The industry died out due to missionary influence and has been revived only recently. About fourteen types of kava now grow in Hawaii.

When kava was in its heyday in the 1800s, Hawaiians had a curious custom—drinking large amounts of kava to purposely induce the scaly skin condition caused by the herb's overconsumption. After the scales fell off, the Hawaiians' skin was soft and smooth—a "molting" experience they relished.

In the nineteenth century, kava drinking became a sacred, esteemed custom in Hawaii. With the exception of water and coconut milk, no other beverage was known. Chiefs drank it before meals, farmers and fishermen used it to relax, and kahunas employed it in numerous rituals.

Although most exported kava is grown on Fiji and Vanuatu, Hawaii is now taking the export market by storm. Hawaiian kava farmers claim they can grow kava in half the time it takes on other South Sea islands, due to Hawaii's fertile growing conditions and tropical climate. Also, there are fewer shipping and handling problems associated with Hawaiian kava than there are with the rather isolated islands of Fiji and Vanuatu.

Demand for kava has soared so much recently that residents have gone into Hawaiian forests and dug it out of the wild—a practice being discouraged in favor of commercialized kava farming.

Hawaii's kava industry looks bright. Dried kava root powder is also sold in many Hawaiian country stores. The Hawaii Kava Growers Association has been formed to take advantage of the burgeoning kava market, and in

May 1997 the first annual international botanical conference on kava was held on the Big Island.

TAHITI

Located about 2,800 miles southeast of Hawaii, Tahiti is a tropical paradise of coconut groves, mountains, reefs, rocky coastlines, and brown/black beaches of volcanic origin. For tourists, there is probably more to see and do on Tahiti than anywhere in the South Pacific, with the exception of Hawaii.

Researchers believe kava may have been brought to Tahiti in the 1700s—much later than it was introduced to other regions of the South Pacific. In those days, chiefs were the only people to imbibe kava. In the 1800s not much was cultivated, largely due to missionary influence. There are possibly fifteen types of kava growing on Tahiti today.

In days gone by, Tahitians classified their kava according to its physiological effects, whereas other island cultures classified it by its physical appearance or potency, as Fijians do today. For example, one type of Tahitian kava has been dubbed *avini-ute,* meaning "pleasure," for its aphrodisiac properties.

AMERICAN SAMOA

Following a colonial dispute in 1899, the land of Samoa was divided in two to form American Samoa and Western Samoa. Draw a triangle from Hawaii to New Zealand to Tahiti, and both Samoas will be squarely in the middle.

A United States territory composed of seven islands, American Samoa is a land of majestic cliffs, beaches, and coral reefs—yet quite Americanized in its towns and villages. Seven kinds of kava grow in American Samoa, and the territory's official seal bears a picture of a kava bowl.

This bowl is traditionally used during kava ceremonies, one of the formal rituals still practiced in Samoan society today.

Though anthropological research proves otherwise, Samoans take credit for spreading the use of kava to other South Sea islands. Legend has it that a Samoan maiden observed a rat falling asleep after chewing on the plant. Consequently, she began using the plant as currency on other islands, in exchange for hens. And kava thus spread from island to island.

For more than three decades, American Samoans living in Hawaii have celebrated Flag Day Festival, which commemorates the establishment of American Samoa as a United States territory. The festival lasts eight days, and its purpose is to build pride in Samoan culture and teach children about Samoan traditions. Among the festival events is a traditional kava ceremony.

WESTERN SAMOA

Made up of four inhabited and five uninhabited islands, Western Samoa is slightly larger than the state of Rhode Island. Its terrain is blessed with rainforest-covered mountains, verdant plains, and calm, reef-protected shores. Although considered by the United Nations one of the world's least developed nations, Western Samoa is experiencing an upswing in tourism, which should help its ailing economy.

Seven varieties of kava grow in Western Samoa. The country's kava ceremonies are quite formal and private, usually held at important meetings of the *matai,* the heads of extended family groups. Visitors normally do not attend the ceremonies as they might in Fiji and Tonga. The kava is prepared by a *taupou,* who in more ancient times was the carefully guarded virgin daughter of a high chief, a ceremonial princess bedecked in feathers and a whale-tooth necklace. Today a taupou still prepares the kava for royal ceremonies, although she may be married and have children.

THE KINGDOM OF TONGA

The Kingdom of Tonga is the oldest and last remaining monarchy in Polynesia and one of the few countries in the world that has never been colonized by a European power. Comprising 170 islands (36 of them inhabited), it is a country of coastal cliffs, charming villages, and lovely waterways.

Eight types of kava are grown on Tonga, and kava-drinking sessions are usually accompanied by lively Polynesian singing, dancing, and instrument playing. These sessions are called "kava circles" and are organized to raise money for Tongan people in need. A woman dances in the midst of a circle of people drinking kava, and the drinkers throw dollar bills at her. Most of the money is collected by the kava-circle organizers and given to needy Tongans, who might use it for medical care, education, and transportation. Kava circles may raise as much as $2,000 a night.

All over Tonga, there are numerous kava clubs, open on Friday nights only. Visitors are welcome, and you can get to a club by asking any taxi driver for a ride.

Tonga is largely a Christian nation, and kava is often a part of religious services. A stem of kava might be presented to a church official during the worship service, and some churches hold kava circles before church. Methodist congregations frequently organize church-sponsored kava clubs to encourage young men to drink kava rather than alcohol.

POHNPEI

Nicknamed the "Garden Island" for its lush, tropical scenery, Pohnpei is located about halfway between Honolulu and Manila. It is the capital of the Federated States of Micronesia (FSM) and has jurisdiction over the islands of Guam, Chuck, Yap, Kosare, and Majero. The FSM is a territory of the United States.

Pohnpei is known for its magnificent beaches, cascading mountain streams, and varied plant life. Most fascinating of all are the ruins of Nan Madol, an ancient city erected in A.D. 500 and notable for its Venice-like canals and ancient stone towers and bridges. The city was built with basalt, which is probably the heaviest rock on earth, and archaeologists are puzzled about how such a small population of ancient peoples (about 25,000) could lift and transport such heavy stones. Legend has it that the people drank kava, which endowed them with superhuman strength!

Two varieties of kava are grown in Pohnpei. Called *sakau,* Pohnpei kava is consumed during meetings among leaders and as a social drink. The island has several sakau bars where visitors can join the locals in drinking a round or two.

Curiously, kava drinking has been incorporated into Roman Catholic church services. Where once natives would bring kava to ruling chiefs to ask for forgiveness, they now offer their kava to God during confession and as their plea for forgiveness. Representing God, the priest drinks the kava as part of the worship service.

THE KAVA CEREMONY

Clearly, kava is a deeply ingrained fixture in island life and social order, not only used socially but ceremonially as well. There are several types of kava ceremonies performed in the South Pacific, and the grandeur of the ceremony often depends on the occasion. One type of ceremony is quite formal—the "full ceremony" or "high kava," as it is called in Fiji, and it is used to welcome honored and distinguished visitors. Another type of ceremony is strictly administrative, held prior to conducting tribal business. There are informal ceremonies and healing ceremonies as well.

All of these ceremonies have various types of paraphernalia associated with kava drinking—utensils that are considered as sacred as the kava itself:

The Pounders. In most places, kava root is no longer chewed. Instead, it is pounded or ground. The preparer places the kava on a kava board or in a kava bowl and mashes the root, using a makeshift mortar such as a piece of wood or metal pipe. For use in kava bars, the root is ground in meat grinders, by power mulchers, or in mechanical pulverizers.

The Kava Board. As noted above, islanders sometimes pound their kava on special wooden boards, which they consider to be treasured possessions.

The Kava Bowl. The ground or mashed kava root is prepared in a wooden, canoe-shaped bowl (*kanoa* in Hawaii and *tanoa* in other parts of Oceania). These are usually cut from a solid section of tree and range in size from smaller bowls adequate for a family to very large bowls used in ceremonies. Archaeologists believe that wooden kava bowls came into use only about four to five hundred years ago. In more ancient times, pottery bowls were used.

Kava bowls usually have legs, and some legs are those of carved human figures. The bowls were often given as gifts. In his journal (January 1778), Captain Cook reported that a Hawaiian chief gave a kava bowl to Captain Clerke, a seaman on all three of Cook's expeditions: ". . . in return he gave him a large Cava bowl, that was supported by carved men, neither ill designed nor executed. Cava or Ava Ava, as it is called at Otahiete is prepared and drank here as at the other islands."

The Strainer. Water from a flask (often a hollowed-out coconut shell) is poured over the mashed root and then passed through a strainer to filter out the solid matter. Strainers are made from various substances including banana stems, bark from hibiscus plants, coconut leaves, and handkerchiefs or mesh cloth. *Aibo* is the Fijian term for "strainer," and in Samoa, it is called *tau tava*.

The Drinking Cups. The drinking cup is usually a hollowed-out half-coconut shell. It is typically scraped smooth on the inside and out, and some cups may have a handle made by woven coconut fiber threaded through holes in the cup. In ancient times, some islanders drank from wooden cups, pottery cups, and even human skulls, according to archaeological records. Today, in towns, kava is often served in glasses.

Although ceremonies vary from land to land, they follow a similar pattern and order. In a formal ceremony, the visiting dignitaries are seated atop a raised platform along with other honored guests, the ruling chief, and his party. Dressed in ceremonial garb, islanders (usually men) arrive, carrying the kava bowl, which they place on pine mats strewn across the platform. Kava is put in the bowl and water poured over it. A kava-maker begins to knead the kava through a strainer until it reaches the desired color and consistency. Next, a server brings him a cup and holds it over the bowl. The kava-maker squeezes the liquid into the cup, and the server offers it to the honored visitor. The guest holds the cup with both hands and drinks it down. If the guest empties the cup, everyone chants *maca,* which means "it is empty," and they clap three times. Clapping is a holdover custom from ancient times, when it was believed to awaken supernatural spirits. The next cup is given to the chief, and the remaining kava drinkers are served according to their rank.

Dignitaries who have taken part in formal kava ceremonies include President and Mrs. Lyndon Johnson upon their visit to Samoa in October 1965, and Pope John Paul II during a 1986 visit to Samoa. Hillary Rodham Clinton, during a 1992 presidential-campaign visit to Hawaii, participated in a kava ceremony conducted in her honor by the Samoan community of Oahu. Queen Elizabeth II of Great Britain and her family always drink kava during welcoming ceremonies when they visit Fiji.

There are also administrative ceremonies performed at meetings of village elders, chiefs, nobles, and visiting chiefs before business is discussed. In fact, no tribal business is conducted until after the kava has been prepared, served, and consumed.

At administrative ceremonies, younger men of the village—usually those without titles—cut, wash, pound, and strain the kava. In most of these ceremonies, kava is prepared in a series of different steps. First, the kava-maker strains the kava root by pressing it through a strainer (usually a mesh cloth), wringing out as much liquid as possible, and cleaning the strainer. This process is repeated over and over again until the brew is free of any root fibers. Before the kava is served, one of the chiefs may recite a poem about the mythic origins of kava.

A strict drinking order is followed: the chief is served first, followed by each member of the hierarchy according to rank. Prior to drinking, the ranking chief may pour a little kava on the ground and ask for God's blessing, since many of these islands are today Christian. The last person to drink usually receives the most potent cup, because kavalactones tend to settle on the bottom of the bowl.

Upon finishing the bowl, the chief announces that it is empty, and those assembled express their thanks. A meal may be served, and the chiefs then get down to business.

Kava drinking evokes an atmosphere of sociability that is conducive to resolving conflicts, peaceably settling business matters, or consummating business contracts.

Informal kava drinking sessions—kava circles or kava parties—are held for social occasions, family gatherings, or other special events. In Fiji, for example, it is common to see a family gathered around a kava bowl filled with the muddy-colored kava brew and drinking it from half coconut shells. Men often drink kava in nakamals (kava bars), while women may drink it at home. Kava parties are usually held in the early evening and may continue well into the night.

Kava ceremonies of welcome are common in Fiji, too. Women help prepare the kava by laying mats out on the floor and setting out a large hand-carved wooden bowl, about three feet across. One person makes the kava, first grating the root with a knife and forming the gratings into a ball. Water is added, and the kava-maker kneads the ball to extract the juices. The entire process is overseen by a master of ceremonies, who determines when the drink reaches the proper consistency and then orders the kava-maker to pour.

Kava is also used in healing ceremonies. Many Pacific peoples believe that illnesses are of a supernatural origin, particularly those that can't be observed, such as internal tumors. Thus, people engage the services of healers who are thought to be empowered with *mana* (a supernatural force) that enables them to heal people suffering from supernaturally induced sickness. Healers use kava to help them divine the exact type of illness. On Vanuatu, mediums drink kava before diagnosing a sickness. And in Hawaii, the kahunas figure out the source of a disease by reading the bubbles that form in the kava bowl. A prayer to heal that particular condition is then offered up to the gods. For his work, the healer is paid in kava.

So esteemed in South Sea culture is kava that it is often presented as a gift: to appease an angry chief, offer friendship, settle quarrels among family members, or mark important occasions such as marriages or funerals. Givers often "dress up" their kava by decorating it with other plants, placing kava cuttings in tree stumps, or changing the shape of the kava root.

KAVA CEREMONIES WITH GUESTS AND FRIENDS

You don't have to venture to a remote South Sea isle to take part in a kava ceremony. As a novel way to entertain, have one in the comfort of your own home. In his book *The Magical and Ritual Use of Herbs,* author Richard Alan Miller suggests serving kava in your finest glassware, or in coconut shells, if you have them. Have everyone stand in a circle, and serve your most honored guests first. Then silently, one by one, each guest should drink a small portion of his or her kava in a single gulp. After each person has consumed a serving, announce that the ceremony is over. Serve some light food, and enjoy a pleasant evening of fellowship.

KAVA BARS

In Fiji, Vanuatu, and other island countries, kava drinks are sold in bars, called *nakamals,* much like alcohol is. The bars are usually rough sheds constructed of woven bamboo, iron, and lumber, with a dirt floor. A counter serves as the bar, with benches lining the outer wall. A single kerosene lamp or low wattage bulb near the bar provides the only lighting.

In late afternoon, the bar owner prepares the fresh kava by washing the roots and scraping off the skin. The kava is ground with a meat grinder, mixed with water, and then squeezed through a coarse cloth. By sunset, patrons begin to arrive (always on an empty stomach to experience kava's maximum effect). In some South Pacific countries, women are usually prohibited from buying and drinking kava. This taboo may have originated from beliefs that kava drinking made women sterile.

A kava drink costs about a dollar and is served in a shelled-out coconut-husk half, as is traditional. The customer sits down on one of the benches and swills his kava in one gulp. Two hours after opening, the kava bars are closed and shut down for the evening, and the customers head home.

AMERICAN KAVA BARS?

No equivalent of the true South Pacific kava bar exists in the United States, but there are places that serve up kava concoctions. One is the highly rated Kava Lounge on 605 Hudson Street in New York City. Decorated with fascinating tribal murals and a Polynesian theme, this cozy West Village establishment is a full-service cocktail lounge featuring Australian and New Zealand wines. Plus, it serves Kava Kava Tea and Deep Kava Smoothies.

Another type of Americanized watering hole for kava

is a juice bar. Juice bars, one of the most rapidly growing segments of the food-service industry, serve fresh-squeezed fruit and vegetable juices, plus "smoothies"—frothy blends of juice, fruit, or yogurt fortified with protein powders, bee pollen, algae, herbs, and other nutrients—and kava.

At the Health Hut, a juice bar on the campus of Miami University in Oxford, Ohio, kava has become the single most popular drink, according to *The Miami Student Online.* The powdered root is mixed in a blender with water and olive oil and costs a dollar for one three-ounce shot. It takes about three of these shots to feel kava's relaxing effects, which last about an hour or two.

You can usually find kava served in major cities, too. A juice bar in Boston called South End Naturals concocts a fresh-fruit beverage pleasantly laced with kava. Other juice drinks on the menu are infused with ginseng, wheat grass, bee pollen, or yohimbe (an herb reputed to increase sexual potency in men).

An alternative to juice bars is the "tonic bar." One of the most popular and well publicized of these is Elixr Tonics & Teas in Los Angeles, a tea salon and retail shop that serves teas and "tonics," herbal drinks designed to restore vitality and well-being. You can sip while relaxing on an outdoor patio overlooking an herb garden.

Elixr is a favorite watering hole for celebrities. The tonic bar has a boutique, a small reference library, a computer database with information on more than 1,200 herbs, formulas, and diseases, and it sells an array of healthy products. One of these is Sweet Slumber Tonic, an herbal blend of kava, passionflower, valerian, and other herbs. You can order it and other Elixr products by accessing the shop's web page at www.elixirnet.com.

Los Angeles is also home to the one and only Fiji club

in California—the Kava Klub, located in Los Angeles county within a sixty-mile radius of Los Angeles International Airport. The restaurant has kava-and-curry nights and features Pacific and Fijian music and entertainment. There is also a Tongan kava club in San Bruno, California, just south of San Francisco.

Each year in Santa Monica, there's the popular Asian Night Market, usually held in August. It features food and entertainment from the cultures of China, Japan, Thailand, Korea, Fiji, Vietnam, Malaysia, Singapore, and the Philippines. One of the newest attractions is a booth that serves kava.

Additionally, kava parties may be a new trend in entertainment. In 1998 a group in Provo, Utah, held a spring-break kava party, promoted as two nights of kava drinking, music, and flashing lights.

If you want to locate restaurants in the United States that serve up South Pacific fare or learn more about how to sample kava while traveling, consult any dining or travel guide.

CHAPTER 4

Kava Experiences

So—what is kava *really* like?

Answer: It depends! If you travel to Vanuatu, Fiji, or Tonga, where the natural kava is served, you could swill down quite a potent dose and end up feeling no pain.

People have been recounting their kava experiences since the plant was first discovered by Westerners during expeditions to the South Pacific. Here are several historical accounts, dating from the 1800s, of the effects of kava brewed from fresh plants:

"Copious draughts cause a dizziness and a horribly distorted countenance. They lose the use of their limbs and fall and roll about on the ground until the stupefaction wears away."

"A well-prepared kava kava potion, drunk in small quantities produces only pleasant changes in behavior. It is therefore a slightly stimulating drink which helps relieve great fatigue. It relaxes the body after strenuous efforts, clarifies the mind and sharpens the mental faculties. Kava soothes temperaments."

"While tramping in the woods I have often moistened my tongue with a piece of awa chipped from some root, and experienced relief from thirst by its pleasant, cooling, aromatic, numbing effect in the mucous membrane of the tongue."

"The head is affected pleasantly; you feel friendly, not beer sentimental; you cannot hate with kava in you. Kava quiets the mind; the world gains no new color or rose tint; it fits in its place and in one easily understandable whole."

A KINDER, GENTLER KAVA?

On the other hand, try the more Americanized versions—capsules, extracts, or powder—and the effects aren't so pronounced. In fact, you may feel nothing at all. Kava capsules, for example, work behind the scenes to take the edge off when you're under stress. Case in point: A thirty-nine-year-old lab technician, who was suffering as a result of severe daily job pressures, decided to participate in a four-week clinical study on stress sponsored by Natrol, Inc., the makers of Kavatrol. After four weeks of taking Kavatrol as recommended, she experienced dramatic improvement: "I love this stuff," she said. "I'm less stressed-out, I'm a lot calmer, I have more fun, and I'm not worried about things. It works wonders for PMS, too." She added that she takes kava for better sleep, for headaches and gastric problems. Nor did the herb affect her manual dexterity—a necessary skill for her occupation.

After reporting on the kava trend in the United States, some staffers at *Forbes Magazine* decided to try one of the kava products. Their consensus: The product produced "mild cheerfulness and no discernible calm."

Keep in mind that each person responds differently to

kava. Plus, the potency of kava still varies from product to product, even though it's not the fresh stuff. Some people say they feel a "buzz," others feel nothing at all. An "unexplainable" feeling is another way kava's effects have been described.

In certain news groups on the Internet, kava use is hotly debated. Here's a sampling of comments, good and bad, about kava:

"Kava kava is a wonderful psychoactive herb. Calming, euphoric, but not sedating."

"There were some capsules I'd gotten that contained an extract of kava kava, and we took them on a mostly empty stomach. The evening was pleasant . . . it felt like we were moving slower, or in a slightly different reality than other people. This wasn't a bad thing, but was strange and took getting used to."

"It has helped me immensely with my problems with depression, anxiety, and insomnia, and it feels great."

"Avoid kava kava like the plague. The Polynesians may be used to it. Unless you are a South Pacific islander, don't touch it!"

"Like everything else, too much kava can hurt you both physically and possibly mentally. I personally do not like the taste. The muddy taste . . . but these characteristics are quickly overcome by an elated feeling of flying free . . . a good feeling!"

"It takes the edge off and produces a feeling of calmness."

"Unlike many drugs and intoxicants, kava makes the mind stay very clear. You know what is going on around you. At the same time, you're apt to feel very loving, with an urge to hug strangers. A sociable drink, kava may make you laugh, too."

"There is a feeling of serenity and a dissipation of anxiety."

"By the time I'd finished [drinking kava], I was more relaxed than I can manage to do to myself with all my yoga."

"There is relaxation, loss of inhibition, happiness, elation, euphoria, contentment . . . all without a hangover."

"And where alcohol can make many people belligerent, kava produces no such effect. In fact, villagers rely on it to resolve peacefully their disputes. What's more, because the arms and limbs become so heavy and limp after drinking it, it would be difficult for two kava drinkers to get into a fight."

"Overconsumption makes the limbs feel heavy and unsteady and you can become inebriated and exhausted."

Some people who have tried kava-root powder say the most noticeable effect is a numbing of the mucus membranes just inside the mouth—a feeling that is similar to Novocain. For some, that is the only feeling experienced—no sedation or intoxication. In others, it can take several days of use before anything is felt at all.

Others report that kava drinking produces very vivid dreams and restful sleep.

Most people who have sampled the drink do agree that its taste is very unpleasant. "Dishwater," "muddy water," "gross," "licoricelike bitter," "each sip gets worse" are typical reactions to kava's bad taste.

TRYING KAVA

As part of the research for this book, I felt compelled to try some of the kava products available. What effects did they have? Were they in the least way comparable to what I had read about the strength of the native brew? I shy away from substances that affect the mind in any altering way—I don't even take medicinal drugs, unless I can help it—thus, I felt a little odd about experimenting. Still, I had to be familiar with the effects of a natural product that has the potential to help millions of anxiety sufferers and stressed-out people—a product with potential addictive or harmful side effects.

My first experiment was conducted with kava capsules. I took four (that's double the recommendation) in the late morning, on an empty stomach. For about an hour I felt rather relaxed.

I decided to try a kava-root-extract product next. The promotional material that accompanied my order noted that this product was a concentrated alcohol that could be used straight from the dropper or added to hot water for a "delightful tea that lifts the spirit and calms the body." I decided to sample the kava straight from the dropper. The suggested use was two to five dropperfuls. So I squirted five dropperfuls of the muddy-colored liquid straight into my mouth. Almost immediately, there was a slight numbing sensation on my tongue and all around the inside of my mouth. It was an unusual feeling, but not unlike Novocain. The sensation lasted a full five minutes.

The liquid tasted very bitter, with a tinge of licorice. It left an aftertaste that wore off in about a minute.

Other than the numbing, I experienced no physical effects, nor any psychoactive effects. I found myself in a good mood, however. Admittedly, though, it was Friday afternoon, the end of the workday—which could have accounted for my mood.

That night I also slept more soundly than I had in a long time. Every night, typically between one and three o'clock in the morning, my dog scratches the bedspread, wanting to snuggle in bed with my husband and me. This noise always awakens me. But not after taking the kava. I slept right through the scratching and never woke up once during the night.

The following week, I conducted my third experiment, this time with a cocoa-flavored kava product I had ordered via the Internet. It came packaged in the squarish-type cans that regular cocoa or powdered hot chocolate usually comes in. I pried open the lid and took a whiff of the chocolate-colored powder. It smelled earthy, yet chocolaty. The powder was "ready-to-use"; that is, I didn't have to strain it through a mesh cloth. The directions said to mix one to two (I opted for two) tablespoons in a half cup of cold water. I did so, and the powder dissolved very well, yielding a mocha-colored liquid. The directions also noted that the drink should be taken on an empty stomach. At three o'clock in the afternoon, mine was quite empty.

I swilled the liquid in about three fast gulps, as the instructions directed. It tasted pretty awful—like muddy rainwater, to be sure, or what you might imagine muddy rainwater to taste like. Almost immediately, there was a slight numbing sensation within my mouth, though not as pronounced as what I had felt with the extract. The numbness lasted no more than a minute or two.

Having been skeptical about whether packaged, non-fresh kava could actually produce any physical sensations, I was quite surprised by what happened next. Fifteen minutes after downing the beverage, I began feeling noticeably relaxed. My arms and lower legs were tingling, and the feeling was quite pleasant. This was not a feeling of inebriation or intoxication—just a gentle, soothing experience. In fact, it was quite similar to the endorphin rush you feel following a hard aerobic workout. My mental faculties felt quite sharp. I was very focused.

Also, the kava totally dulled my appetite. I had no desire for food and consequently ate dinner a few hours later than usual.

Then, I took another cup (two tablespoons again) exactly one half hour later, as the South Pacific Islanders customarily do. My lips and mouth became a little more anesthetized than they had been after the first serving—a sensation that lasted only a minute. As if on cue, fifteen minutes after drinking the second cup, the relaxation intensified, but I felt quite slow-moving. In fact, I didn't want to move. I just wanted to sit and enjoy my surroundings (I was lounging on my deck in the backyard, under a canopy of dogwood trees). Although I felt extremely relaxed physically, mentally I was very lucid and focused. I decided that the feeling kava produces is entirely physical and that it appears to sharpen one's mental faculties. Based on my experience, I would call kava "body-altering."

The decision to drink a second cup had not been a good idea. It made me feel slightly nauseous—a feeling that superseded the kava's relaxing effects. If a product happens to be high in dihydrokavain and dihydromethysticum, it may cause nausea and headaches. Of course, it's difficult to know the actual chemical makeup of a kava product. Capsules and extracts are more likely to be standardized and less likely to cause such side effects, whereas dry root kava bought in bulk could vary widely in its concentrations of active components.

The lesson here: Don't drink more than what the manufacturer recommends. At four-thirty in the afternoon, I took two gingerroot capsules to quell my queasiness.

Over the next couple of hours, the relaxation as well as the queasiness gradually dissipated, giving way to a mild drowsiness. I slept very soundly that evening and experienced no aftereffects of my experiment.

My husband, Jeff, tried the brew as well—three tablespoons in cold water (he's much bigger than me). He felt that it didn't taste that bad and he experienced the usual slight numbing in his mouth. As for other sensations, Jeff noted that his legs and arms felt a little rubbery. He, too, had some slight nausea. That night, unlike me, Jeff did not have a restful sleep. Go figure!

Next experiment: The kava product I tried this time required mixing three tablespoons of dry root powder into a cup of cold water, then pouring the mixture into a mesh cloth to strain out particles of root. I used a piece of old hosiery as a strainer. I squeezed the liquid through the mesh of the hosiery into a bowl until there was nothing left but what resembled caked pieces of tan-colored mud.

I drank the tannish liquid in a couple of gulps. It tasted like muddy water with a hint of licorice and cinnamon. This time, I felt no numbing of the mouth or tongue. By this experiment, it was clear to me that kava is rapid-acting. In fifteen minutes, I felt mildly relaxed and slightly mellow. However, these feelings were extremely faint, not pronounced at all, and quite comparable to the mild "endorphin high" often felt following exercise—a very natural, nonnarcotic and nonsedating tranquillity. My slumber that night was quite deep, and I felt great the next morning—energized enough to begin the day with forty-five minutes of a hard aerobic workout.

A week or so later, I sampled a dried kava-root product shipped to me from Hawaii but grown in Fiji. It arrived in a plastic bag labeled with two options for mixing—the traditional method, which involved straining through a sieve or mesh, or the "blender method." Opting for the blender method, I poured two cups of cold water, a teaspoon of olive oil, and two tablespoons of the greenish-brown powder into the blender and blended for two minutes on high, as instructed. The directions stated that the liquid could then be strained, if desired. I decided to swill it down without doing so. This sample tasted truly revolting. I imagine that the taste of this root powder must be close to what the South Sea island natives drink. Again, it tasted like muddy water, but muddy water with lumps in it (I guess I should have strained it). I could not make myself finish the cup. Within seconds my mouth and tongue felt faintly numb—a very subtle numbness. As usual, a sense of relaxation set in after fifteen minutes, with some gentle tingling in my legs and arms. The kava produced a very mild feeling of calm and tranquillity, but without any narcotic or intoxicating fog. This feeling lasted for about two hours.

These experiments were simply personal, and certainly not scientific. In my opinion, kava seems to be an incredible stress-reliever—perfect for trying times when you just can't relax or get rid of health-damaging physical tension. Further, it has the potential to help you endure any situation that makes you jittery: flying in an airplane, meeting tight deadlines, speaking in public, and so forth.

Think of kava as a "stress Band-Aid," though—an emergency way to temporarily ease the crisis until you can resolve it.

For mild cases of anxiety, even mild depression, you may want to try kava—because it's so kind to the body—but get your physician's or psychiatrist's blessing first.

TROUBLE IN PARADISE?

As noted, kava is legal in the United States and elsewhere, and continues to occupy a central place in everyday life in the South Pacific. Taken in moderate dosages for short periods of time, kava has virtually no side effects and is one of the safest herbs around. But like any substance—pharmaceutical or herbal—it can be abused, crossing the line from safe to dangerous.

Kava is raising a ruckus in some parts of the South Pacific. Women and welfare groups, for example, have complained that kava use has turned to abuse, with men binge-drinking kava up to twelve hours a day. There have been numerous outcries from women's groups to limit consumption because of the time men spend drinking kava.

In the island nation of Kiribati, which does not cultivate kava, the Department of Social Welfare says people are spending too much time drinking kava—a problem that is causing the deterioration of family health and welfare. According to the government, some kava drinkers imbibe for forty-eight hours at a stretch.

Heavy, continual kava usage has taken its toll on physical health in some of these communities, according to studies. Take the case of the Aboriginal communities in Australia, where kava, ironically, was introduced to the natives by missionaries in the 1980s as a substitute for alcohol. Prior to that time, they knew nothing about kava. It was gradually much abused, with people consuming as much as fifty times the amount typically drunk by South Pacific islanders. This abuse has led to widespread health problems.

One study of Aborigines found that kava users were more likely to complain of poor health and puffy faces, and have scaly rashes and compromised immunity. The findings prompted medical personnel to push for urgent social action to reduce kava consumption in order to improve health in the communities.

Long-term overconsumption of kava produces a skin condition called "kava dermopathy," which has been observed only in South Pacific islanders and Aboriginal peoples. This condition produces scaly, yellow skin and resembles a disease called pellagra, caused by a deficiency of the B-vitamin niacin. Kava dermopathy was originally thought to be a niacin deficiency, but that link has been disproved. Researchers now believe that chronic kava use interferes with cholesterol metabolism and that this leads to kava dermopathy.

In 1988 a team of researchers surveyed the health status of thirty-nine kava users and thirty-four nonusers in a coastal Aboriginal community. They found that very heavy users (with an average consumption of 440 grams a week) were 20 percent underweight, in poor health, and likely to suffer from kava dermopathy. Other serious health problems that turned up among chronic users were liver and kidney disorders; shortness of breath; and abnormalities in red blood cells, lymphocytes, and platelets. It's important to mention, however, that Aboriginal health is generally the absolute worst, compared to other Australian people. These Aborigines may have been in poor health before they ever started drinking kava.

More recently, the medical literature reported an unusual case of a twenty-seven-year-old Aboriginal Australian man who sought medical treatment at a clinic after bingeing on kava. His symptoms included abnormal movements of limbs, trunk, neck, and facial muscles. Also, his tongue writhed involuntarily. Despite these physical problems, his mind was clear. Doctors administered diazepam (Valium) intravenously, and within twelve hours he had returned to normal. A battery of medical tests, including a brain scan, could find nothing wrong with the man. He didn't drink alcohol and was in good health between kava binges. The doctors concluded that his heavy kava consumption had brought on these severe neurological problems.

The problems with kava drinking in Aboriginal communities has reached such proportions that the government there is looking for ways to control and restrict kava usage. At least one government official has called for a temporary ban on kava.

In the city of Suva, the capital of Fiji, it is rumored that the cable and wireless operators drink kava on the job, making it difficult to place long distance phone calls!

BACK IN THE USA

In the United States kava abuse has raised some concern, too. In the spring of 1997, law enforcement officers in California and Utah pulled over drivers who where weaving in and out of traffic—not because they were drunk on alcohol but because they were intoxicated from kava. In fact, in one arrest and conviction made in Utah, the motorist had consumed sixteen cups of a kava drink (the usual serving is one or two cups).

Moreover, the California Highway Patrol has warned that kava, "when combined with driving, becomes an extreme hazard to the motoring public." A vehicle fatality or serious illness caused by kava intoxication or use could immediately initiate tight regulation of the herb.

Kava has made the news elsewhere. In 1997 kava was falsely accused of causing some severe reactions at a New Year's Eve party held at the Olympic Auditorium in Los Angeles. About fifty party-goers got sick, experiencing

dizziness, nausea, shortness of breath, and respiratory failure, after ingesting a product called fX, which was supposedly formulated with kava. Forty-two people were
later hospitalized, and a seventeen-year-old suffered a
heart attack.

The American Botanical Council in Austin, Texas, had
samples of fX analyzed by an independent lab in Denver.
The results revealed that the product contained some caffeine and a toxic chemical known as butanedoil—but no
kava.

A criminal investigation ensued, and police later discovered that the lab that formulated fX for its manufacturer had been unable to obtain any kava and instead
substituted butanedoil—an act of mislabeling that is a
felony violation of the United States Food, Drug, and
Cosmetic Act. Used as an industrial solvent, butanedoil
acts on the central nervous system and is harmful if swal-
lowed. Two owners of the lab were convicted for the
crime. One spent three months in a community drug
treatment center; the other was sentenced to two years of
supervised probation. Both had to pay $2,000 fines.

TRYING KAVA FOR YOURSELF

There are few things in this world without controversy,
including kava and other natural supplements. Chances
are you'll continue to hear more about kava in the future—pros and cons. But the bottom line is this: Kava is
a natural medicine, and natural medicine is fast becoming
a health care option. The final decision on whether to use
kava is up to you. And that's as it should be. You must
take responsibility for your own physical and mental

health. But remember that kava, like anything else, carries with it the potential for abuse. Use it wisely, with common sense, and always check with your physician or health care provider first.

CHAPTER 5

The Kick
That Kava Gives

In the sixties, LSD-guru Timothy Leary, Ph.D., who coined the term "turn on, tune in, drop out," conducted various experiments with a number of psychoactive drugs while employed in the psychology department at Harvard University. During this period he ordered some samples from a laboratory in Canada. These samples included: ibogaine, a drug thought to help treat drug addiction that comes from a West African shrub called *Tabernanthe Iboga;* psilocine, a synthetic version of the hallucinogen (psilocybin) found in the psilocybe mushroom cultivated in Mexico; bufotenine, a synthetic version of a psychoactive agent isolated from the venom of a certain species of toad; and—you guessed it—kava, in the form of an alcohol extract!

In a letter to Leary, the laboratory noted that the active ingredient in kava was unknown. Further, the letter stated: "When undertaking your clinical work, we cannot stress this strongly enough that medical observers be present. This applies particularly to research with ibogaine and kava kava extract whose pharmacological properties are not too well established."

Fascinating! Of course, more than thirty years later we know plenty about kava and its effects.

EARLY KAVA SCIENCE

Kava has a fascinating scientific and therapeutic history. A pharmacist named G. Cuzent, serving in the French navy in 1857, is generally credited as the first person to isolate a component from kava roots—a crystalline substance he named "kavahine." Cuzent may also have been the first person to have created actual kava supplements. He formulated some kava-based pills, an oleoresin (a preparation of oil that would hold the resinous portion of kava in solution), an alcohol extract, and a syrup.

In 1860 a scientist named M. Gobley isolated a chemical he called "methysticin." Some scientists today point out that Cuzent's kavain and Gobley's methysticin are one in the same. The substance was officially named "methysticin."

Interest continued to accelerate, and more chemicals from kava were isolated, analyzed, and named. In 1874 two scientists, E. Nölting and A. Kopp, isolated another substance from kava; it was named "yangonin" in 1886 by another kava scientist, Lewin. By the end of the nineteenth century, various kava formulations could be purchased in herbal shops in Germany.

As the twentieth century began, activity into the scientific analysis of kava was brisk, and more chemicals in kava were discovered. In 1908 E. Winzheimer isolated dihydromethysticin, which is responsible for kava's tranquilizing effects. Between 1913 and 1933, two other chemicals were discovered, kavain and dihydrokavain. Later scientific experiments in the 1960s revealed that kavain was the chemical responsible for kava's anesthetic effect. In fact, its numbing effect on the surface of tissues is equal to that of cocaine but lasts longer. Yet unlike cocaine, kavain is not toxic to tissues.

In the 1900s kava and kava-based remedies were well-established medicines. They were listed in the Britain Pharmacopoeia, sold in European dispensaries as sedatives and as medicines to counter low blood pressure, and found in the United States Dispensatory (a reference on plants and drugs first published in 1833) as a remedy for irritations of the bladder and reproductive organs. In 1950, in the United States, kava was a bona fide medicine used to treat gonorrhea and nervous conditions, marketed under the trade names Gonosan and Neurocardin, respectively.

By the early 1960s more constituents in kava had been identified, and these included desmethoxy yangonin; 5,6-dehydromethysticin, 11-methoxyyangonin, and 11-methoxynoryangonin. Collectively, all the chemical constituents found in kava were termed "kavalactones." Table 1 lists all the known chemicals in kava, along with their properties.

Kavalactones such as kavain and methysticin can now be synthesized in the lab. However, the synthetic versions do not produce the same effects as the natural product. Also, the various compounds in kava work best synergistically—in other words, not by themselves in isolation, but rather as a team.

FASCINATING FIRST EXPERIMENTS

The earliest scientific experiment on the effects of kava was conducted in the 1800s. L. Lewin, who had named yangonin, injected the resin of the plant into frogs and found that it paralyzed the animals. He did the same to pigeons and sparrows; the injection sedated the birds so much that they were unable to fly. Lewin continued his experiments with cats, which after being injected with kava resin fell into a deep slumber.

By 1924 a scientist by the name of K. Schübel noted that kava resin did indeed produce sleep and could temporarily paralyze sensory nerves and smooth muscles. In experiments with frog hearts, Schübel was the first to confirm that the effects of kava extract were strengthened by the addition of human saliva. He speculated that pytalin, the starch-dissolving enzyme in saliva, released the resinous compounds from the root to yield a more potent extract.

In 1938 an investigator named A. G. Van Veen found that kava's effects could be further enhanced if the extract was put into a lecithin/water emulsion. (Lecithin is a fat found in cells and nerve membranes; in egg yolk, soybeans, and corn; and as an essential constituent of animal and vegetable cells. It helps process cholesterol in the body.) Recent investigations have validated Van Veen's finding. The presence of fats and oils does assist in the absorption and use of kavalactones by the body, thus inducing a stronger effect.

The era of modern kava research was ushered in just after World War II at Freiburg University in southern Germany, with experiments led by H. J. Meyer and his colleagues. During the 1950s and 1960s, his research team became the first to document the vast physiological effects of kavalactones. For example, they confirmed that kavalactones: (1) produce a relaxant effect (particularly dihydromethysticin); (2) work as an analgesic or pain reliever (dihydrokavain and dihydromethysticin are the most powerful in this regard); (3) relax the muscles as effectively as the drugs phenobarbital, pyrimidine, and diphenyhydantoin widely used at the time; and (4) have antifungal and antibacterial effects.

MODERN EXPERIMENTS

Kava and its active constituents are so versatile that they work in a number of different ways in the body. They act directly on muscles, interact with various brain chemicals, and influence different parts of the brain. While not all of kava's actions have been pinned down scientifically, it is clear that the herb works in diverse and unique ways.

KAVA AND THE MUSCLES

One of the most noticeable effects of taking kava is mild muscle relaxation. Your limbs may feel a little rubbery, perhaps tingly. What causes these pleasant sensations?

An animal study published in 1983 found that certain constituents in kava suppress the mechanisms that make muscles contract, causing a degree of paralysis. The result is the rather mellow feeling you experience after having some kava.

KAVA AND BRAIN CHEMICALS

The billions of cells in your brain use roughly one hundred "neurotransmitters," hormonal brain chemicals that transmit messages from one nerve cell to another across the gap, or synapse, between the two.

The action of neurotransmitters can be modified by certain drugs such as tranquilizers or antidepressants to produce the desired change in mood. The drug enters the brain and links up with compatible "receptors," tiny structures mounted on the surface of cells. Receptors are like cellular peepholes that recognize substances and allow their entry into the cells. Once inside cells, the drug intensifies or weakens the action of certain neurotransmitters, affecting behavior.

There are four neurotransmitters that may be influenced by kava and its active kavalactones:

GABA. Technically known as gamma-aminobutyric acid, GABA is the brain's natural tranquilizer. Made from the amino acid glutamine, GABA is an "inhibitory" neurotransmitter. It prevents anxiety messages from being transmitted from nerve cell to nerve cell. When the brain doesn't produce enough GABA, depression, anxiety, and panic attacks can result. According to an animal study conducted in 1994, kava enters brain cells through GABA receptors, then possibly stimulates GABA inside cells, producing more GABA in the brain and thus causing relaxation and sedation. Drugs like Valium do the same thing.

Dopamine. Found in every nook and cranny in the brain, dopamine's chief function in the body is to initiate normal muscle movement. Kava, however, may partly block the action of dopamine in the brain—with side effects occurring in susceptible people. Several years ago a group of German doctors treated four patients who had symptoms of a dopamine system gone awry—abnormal muscle spasms and contortions. What all patients had in common was that they had been taking some form of kava preparation. A few had been taking other drugs, too.

The first case was of a twenty-eight-year-old man who had been taking medication for anxiety. He also had a history of abnormal muscle spasms. He tried the kava extract Laitan, but began having neck spasms ninety minutes after taking a dose. This reaction subsided on its own within forty minutes.

The second case was of a twenty-two-year-old woman taking Laitan for anxiety and nervousness. Four hours after her first dose, her tongue started jerking, her neck went into spasms, and her trunk started twisting—all involuntarily. Doctors gave her a drug to ease the spasms, and she recovered.

A similar reaction occurred in a sixty-three-year-old woman taking the kava preparation Kavasporal for anxiety. She was treated with a spasm-relieving drug as well. Both women denied taking other drugs in the months prior to the attack.

The fourth case involved a seventy-six-year-old woman suffering from Parkinson's disease. For eight years, she had been treated with levodopa, a drug given to relieve the muscle stiffness, tremor, and weakness caused by Parkinson's disease. Still, spells of muscle spasms and jerking movements were increasing. Her general practitioner prescribed Kavasporal for inner tension. But within ten days, her spells lasted longer and were more frequent. She discontinued taking Kavasporal, and the intensity of the spells was subdued.

The doctors cautioned that in some people (particularly the elderly) kava extracts may negatively influence the brain systems that affect bodily movement, due to their possible interference with dopamine. These cases appear to be extremely rare though they do indicate that kava extracts have some effect on dopamine. Laitan and Kavasporal are available in Europe. For more information on both preparations, see chapter 14.

Serotonin. A "happiness neurotransmitter," serotonin is associated with tranquillity, calm, and emotional well-being. Low levels may increase the risk for depression or suicide. Based on experiments with animals, some scientists believe that kava constituents may influence a serotonin receptor that is involved in relieving anxiety.

Norepinephrine. As one of the brain's "alert" neurotransmitters, norepinephrine prepares you for action in threatening situations. It also helps to regulate blood pressure and to maintain your ability to concentrate. The kavalactone, kavain, appears to block the uptake of norepinephrine by brain cells, according to a 1997 animal study. The scientists who conducted the experiment feel that this blockade may somehow be responsible for kava's effects on the mind.

KAVA AND THE LIMBIC SYSTEM

Kava and its active kavalactones work on a fascinating region of the brain known as the limbic system. The limbic system is actually a group of interdependent structures involved in regulating blood pressure, heart rate, body temperature, appetite, thirst, sleep, emotions, hormones, and many other body functions.

Within the limbic system is a cluster of cells about the size of a chickpea called the amygdala. The term, derived from the Greek word for almond, describes the organ's shape. As with most structures in the brain, there are two amygdalae—one in the left side of your brain and one in the right.

The amygdala is involved in mood and emotions, particularly the acquisition and expression of fear and anxiety. It also helps you vividly recall emotionally charged events from your past.

More specifically, the amygdala is like an alarm center in your brain. It takes input from your senses and orchestrates your reaction to it. Suppose you're walking down a dark alley and see a man coming toward you, wielding a knife. Your heart starts beating rapidly, your facial expression contorts into a look of panic, and you scream.

Each of these responses—the rapid heartbeat, the facial expression, the flight—was activated by the amygdala the instant it received visual cues signaling danger. Put another way, the amygdala interprets the significance of a threatening situation, then organizes your emotional and bodily response to that threat. It communicates with other regions of the brain, particularly those that control breathing, heart rate, the release of hormones, etc.

In a laboratory, when scientists introduce a cat into the lab's rat habitat, the rats' blood pressure and heart rate instinctively soar. But remove the amygdala from the rats' brains, and they impassively ignore the cat.

Of course, no such scientific experiment could ever be performed on people. However, in 1993 a team of neuroscientists at the University of Iowa College of Medicine had a rare opportunity to study how this tiny organ functions. They tested a patient whose right and left amygdala had been damaged by disease. Although her memory and emotions were intact, her fear response was not. She was unable to discern—or imitate—facial expressions exhibiting fear.

Additionally, scientists speculate that the amygdala may be implicated in panic disorders. In a 1978 experiment, researchers electrically stimulated the amygdala in humans, and this produced the physical and emotional symptoms of a panic attack. Other experiments using sophisticated brain scans have revealed that increased blood flow to the amygdala stimulates it, triggering panic attacks or causing depression.

In further studies in which scientists have electrically stimulated the amygdala, people report feeling anxiety, fear, depression, malaise—and are even able to recollect nightmarish episodes from their past in vivid detail.

There's more: A 1997 study found that abnormally high glucose metabolism in the amygdala may produce depression, too. The chief fuel for brain cells is glucose, also known as blood sugar. In this study, investigators using high-tech scanners peered into the brains of depressed patients and confirmed that there was increased glucose metabolism in the amygdala. In other words, the organ was using up lots of blood sugar.

Dr. Wayne Drevets, associate professor of psychiatry and radiology at the University of Pittsburgh Medical Center, and leader of the study, noted that the research also linked abnormal amygdala metabolism with elevated cortisol in depression. Cortisol is a stress hormone—one that the bodies of depressed people overproduce.

"There's a sort of chemical cascade in the body that's responsible for releasing cortisol," Dr. Drevets stated in a press release. "That cascade is called the hypothalamic-pituitary-adrenal axis. That axis is overly active in depression, and our study is the first to suggest that the overactive amygdala might be the explanation for this effect."

The bottom line of all of this fascinating research is that an overactive, overstimulated amygdala appears to account for anxiety, panic attacks, depression, and depression with symptoms of anxiety. Kava is believed to calm an overactive amygdala.

The amygdala is a principal site of activity for the biologically active kavalactones in kava—as well as for prescription tranquilizers (particularly the class of antianxiety drugs known as benzodiazepines).

As noted above, brain cells have little structures known as "receptors" that recognize and allow entry through the cell wall. Benzodiazepine receptors, for example, recognize benzodiazepines. It just so happens that the cells in the amygdala have more benzodiazepine receptors than anywhere else in the brain. Which means that the amygdala is an important place for benzodiazepines to do their work.

But even though antianxiety drugs and antidepressants have helped many people, their worrisome side effects and the problems associated with withdrawal are medically risky, sometimes life-threatening. What we now know about kava, however, suggests that it may treat anxiety disorders, and possibly depression, more effectively than benzodiazepines and certainly without the toxicity and withdrawal symptoms.

TABLE I

Chemical Constituents of Kava

Constituents	Major Biological Activities
Benzoic Acid	Antifungal, antiseptic, diuretic, expectorant
Cinnamic Acid	Anesthetic, antibacterial, antifungal, laxative
Cinnamylidenacetol	None
Desmethoxyyangonin	None
*Dihydrokavain	Anesthetic, anti-inflammatory, fever-reducer, muscle-relaxant, sedative
Dihydrokavain-5-OL	None
*Dihydromethysticin	Anesthetic, anti-inflammatory, fever-reducer, CNS-depressant, muscle relaxant, sedative
5-Dihydroyangonin	None
Dimethoxydihydrokavain	None
Flavokavain-A	None
Flavokavain-B	None
Flavokavain-C	None
11-Hydroxy-12-methoxydihydrokavain	None
*Kavain	Anesthetic, anti-inflammatory, fever-reducer, antiseptic, muscle relaxant, tranquilizer
Kavainic-Acid	None
3,4-(Methylene-dioxy) Cinnamylidenacetol	None
11-Methoxynoryangonin	None

11-Methoxyyangonin	None
*Methysticin	Anesthetic, anti-inflammatory, antipyretic, muscle relaxant
Pipermethystine (a major constituent of the leaves)	None
5,6,7,8-Tetrahydroyangonin	None
*Yangonin	Anesthetic, anti-inflammatory, fever-reducer, antibacterial, muscle relaxant

*These are considered the "major kavalactones" because they account for more than 96 percent of extracted kava. The rest are termed "minor kavalactones."

CHAPTER 6

Kava:

Nature's Stress Cure

Most of us think of stress as missing deadlines, blowing a sales call, failing a test, arguing with a spouse, or losing a loved one. But in medical lingo, stress is a series of physiological reactions to events. When we're faced with a real or perceived threat, stress prepares our bodies to run from or contend with the situation. This sets off a cascade of biochemical events, including a surge of hormones, to help your body defend itself. Your muscles tense, your stomach knots up, your heart races, or your palms sweat—reactions that are all part of this series of events.

Under normal conditions, these stress reactions protect us from danger, but if stress goes unresolved and becomes chronic, there's trouble. In fact, medical experts estimate that stress accounts for more than 90 percent of all illnesses and trips to the doctor.

Just how damaging is chronic stress to health? Here's a glimpse into what happens physiologically when stress goes unresolved.

1. Stress gets under your skin. Hives, acne, itching, eczema, and other common skin disorders are caused or aggravated by chronic stress.

2. Stress produces tension headaches. The most common of all headaches, tension headaches, occur when the muscles surrounding your skull go into painful spasms. Blood vessels in the scalp may enlarge, too. Though not life-threatening, tension headaches are often a clear sign that you are depressed or under pressure. If they persist, your body may be warning you to change your lifestyle.

3. Stress assaults your immune system. When you're persistently stressed-out or depressed, your adrenal glands churn out cortisol and adrenaline, two emergency hormones. Normally these hormones help us handle stress. But if that stress is chronic, these hormones stick around. Cortisol, in particular, isn't metabolized well. Plus, it does damage to both the cardiovascular and immune systems.

Your body really takes a beating when hormones work overtime and your immune system begins to wear down, giving way to brittle bones, infections, and even cancer. In a study of bone density among twenty-six women (all in their forties), half the group suffered from depression, while the other half was emotionally stable. The depressed women had higher levels of stress hormones—and the bone density of seventy-year-old women!

Also, according to research from Duke University Medical Center, watching violence on TV or at the movies elevates cortisol, drives up your blood pressure, and raises your heart rate—reactions that promote heart disease and batter your immune system.

4. Unresolved stress may shrink your brain. Researchers studied a group of thirty-eight women—twenty with a history of sexual abuse. Using magnetic resonance imaging (MRI) to peer into their brains, the researchers discovered that in those women who had been sexually abused as children, the hippocampus was smaller than normal. The hippocampus is a seahorse-shaped structure deep within the brain that helps you learn and remember. The researchers speculate that this shrinkage may be caused by prolonged exposure to cortisol and other stress hormones. Thus, stress can make you not only frazzled, but forgetful, too.

5. Stress is a heartbreaker. In a recent study 1,305 healthy men between the ages of forty and ninety were tested on their ability to control anger, then followed for seven years to see who suffered heart attacks. The findings: The men with the shortest fuses had more than triple the risk of nonfatal heart attacks and fatal coronary heart disease, even after the researchers adjusted for smoking and alcohol use.

Many studies in the last twenty years have found that people who exhibit hostile emotions have a much higher rate of heart disease and its warning signs than do people without such hostility. Other studies have found that men who are "self-involved"—in other words, very me-centered—tend to have more extensively blocked arteries (a heart-attack risk) than men who are less self-involved. Self-centered heart patients are also more prone to second heart attacks. Scientists theorize that frequent surges in stress-related chemicals contribute to heart-damaging processes.

Everyday emotions such as tension, frustration, and sadness may trigger myocardial ischemia—lack of oxygen to the heart muscle (which increases the chance of heart attack). This finding comes from a study of fifty-eight male heart patients, who, while being heart-monitored for two days, kept a diary of their activities and moods. The results showed that common emotions nearly doubled the risk of ischemia.

6. Stress breaks down your defenses. In a scientific experiment at Ohio State University, researchers investigated the effects of exam stress on students. The experiment revealed that stress interfered with the function of "natural killer cells," which help the body combat foreign invaders that cause disease. The stress brought on by exams also reduced the body's production of interferon, a type of protein that fights viruses and boosts immunity—your body's armor against illness.

Also, stress unleashes too much nerve growth factor (NGF), a chemical that tacks itself onto disease-fighting cells and prevents them from fighting infections. Up to six hours after they hit the ground, first-time parachute jumpers had NGF levels that were 107 percent higher than nonjumpers, according to one study.

7. Stress aggravates rheumatoid arthritis, a painful immune disease that attacks and inflames the joints and other organs. In response to stress, the pituitary gland (a control center for the body), discharges a hormone called prolactin. It travels to the joints and sets off a chain of events that cause tenderness, pain, and swelling. Rheumatoid arthritis patients under interpersonal stress have higher levels of prolactin than those who are not stressed.

8. Kids who grow up in stressful, conflict-ridden homes tend to be shorter in stature, says a British study. Investigators at London's Royal Free Hospital studied 6,574 British boys and girls born in the same week in 1958 and tracked for nearly forty years as part of a national child development study. Their heights were checked at age seven, and the shortest of the group were singled out for a separate study on the effect of stress on growth. Nearly three hundred of these children came from homes with family conflict, divorce, separation, or desertion. Of these, a third were short in stature, leading the investigators to conclude that there is a link between childhood growth and family conflict.

They speculate that family stress might raise levels of beta-endorphin, a chemical produced by the brain in response to stress. Beta-endorphin curbs the amount of growth hormone (a natural chemical that produces growth in children) released in the body. Other studies on stress in children have found that long-term family conflict interferes with the development of the hippocampus, the part of the brain that deals with learning and memory.

Clearly, stress is hazardous to your health. It is destructive to practically every physiological system. How well you cope with stress makes all the difference in your health and well-being.

A PROVEN STRESS-REDUCER

Kava is truly nature's stress cure—one of the best natural relaxers and tranquilizers around. It helps you manage stress in two important ways. First, it counteracts the physical symptoms of stress, such as pounding heartbeat or tensed muscles. Second, it works biochemically on brain chemicals and on regions of the brain responsible for emotion to produce a calming effect.

Increasingly, people are discovering that kava can get them through the stressful times. When ABC's *20/20* aired a report on kava on June 22, 1998, reporter Perri Peltz featured a seventeen-year-old student under a lot of pressure over classes and schoolwork. His psychologist gave him the okay to take a 120-milligram dose of kava-lactones three times a day. After being on kava, the student said he felt a lot less stressed out, and even his friends noticed his newfound calm.

Stress-relieving benefits like these have now been proven scientifically in the first clinical study ever conducted to measure the effects of kava on the daily hassles of life. Two professors at the Medical College of Virginia at Virginia Commonwealth University—Nirbhay N. Singh, Ph.D. and Cynthia R. Ellis, M.D.—led the landmark study, which was conducted in 1997. From ads in health food stores, pharmacies, supermarkets, as well as referrals from physicians, they recruited sixty subjects between the ages of eighteen and sixty who had elevated levels of daily stress and anxiety. These volunteers were placed in one of two groups, a kava group or a placebo group. The kava product used was Kavatrol, a brand-name product from Natrol, Inc., a California-based manufacturer of nutritional supplements.

Over the course of four weeks, each person took two capsules of kava or of a placebo twice a day. Each dose (two capsules) of the kava product contained 120 milligrams of kavalactones.

The stress level of each volunteer was assessed five times during the study: prior to the start of the study (to obtain a benchmark for comparison purposes), and at weeks one, two, three, and four. Volunteers were assessed in five areas: interpersonal problems, personal competency, cognitive stressors, environmental hassles, and other stressors.

Among the kava-takers, stress significantly declined from week to week in every category, while those in the placebo group showed little change. Additionally, the study found that the longer a person took the kava supplements, the greater the reduction in stress.

The study also examined the potential side effects of

the herb and concluded that it is not addictive, nor do users build up a tolerance to the supplement (meaning they don't need to increase the dose to get an effect).

Dr. Singh has been a pioneer in the use and study of kava. A native of Fiji, he first consumed it forty years ago in a ritual prepared by his father. More than ten years ago, he conducted the first study on the effects of kava on long-term memory. Since then, kava has received increasingly more attention for its stress-reducing and relaxation benefits, and in February 1998, the *Wall Street Journal* said in a major story that "kava is poised to become the next blockbuster herbal remedy."

MORE STRESS CURES

Kava is clearly an important weapon in your anti-stress arsenal. But although taking kava is a gentle, healthy, nonaddictive way to alleviate stress and tension, it is still only a temporary fix. There are really no easy-outs when it comes to stress resolution. Ultimately, you need a comprehensive way to deal with the inevitable, inescapable stress that intrudes on your life. Here are some practical guidelines for handling stress that will help you minimize its potentially damaging health effects.

Fortify yourself nutritionally. Stress robs your body of nutrients. Suppose you're stuck in traffic, and you're late for a meeting. During this entire time, your body is rapidly using up vitamin C, vitamin B complex, and protein. Just a single stressful event takes a huge toll on your nutritional health!

What's a stressed-out body to do? Fortify yourself nutritionally, starting with meals. Make sure you eat at least five servings of fruits and vegetables daily. And with every meal, eat some protein (fish, poultry, lean meats, legumes, or low-fat dairy products). Include several servings of whole grains daily, too.

As important, take a daily multivitamin/mineral antioxidant supplement as nutritional insurance. An amino acid supplement, available in capsules or protein powder, may help, too, although you can get ample amino acids from protein foods. Amino acids, which are protein particles, are sacrificed under stressful conditions. One amino acid in particular, tyrosine, helps build your natural store of adrenaline and assists your body in fighting stress. Tyrosine has also been found to counter stress-related depression. Foods high in tyrosine include almonds, peanuts, cheese, nonfat dried milk, avocados, and bananas. (For more information on tyrosine and other natural tranquilizers, see chapter 14.)

When stressed out, some people binge on junk foods for comfort, or stop eating altogether. Both habits are health damaging and only make things worse. Gobbling up a quart of ice cream after a bad day will only amplify your stress and hurt your self-image. Avoiding food altogether will sap your strength and further wear you down. Try to establish some sensible eating patterns for the good times as well as the bad.

Also, cut down on stress-inducing substances such as caffeine. These can actually trigger the fight-or-flight responses typical of stress attacks, and elevate hormone levels. Avoid or limit your use of alcohol, too, since it acts as a depressant.

Rub it away. There's no doubt about it: Massage is one of the best stress soothers around. It relaxes muscles that have tensed up due to mental strain and anxiety and allows more oxygen and nutrients to reach body cells by improving circulation and blood flow. Plus, studies show that massage releases endorphins (brain chemicals that improve mood). In fact, some massage therapists say some of their clients pop kava prior to the massage. Kava apparently heightens the physical sensations of the massage.

Sweat it out. Exercise, particularly the aerobic type, is one of the most effective ways to dissipate physical and emotional stress. It speeds up the production of feel-good endorphins—thought to be responsible for the pleasurable sensation called the "runner's high" that joggers and marathoners experience. Exercise also relieves the muscular tension brought on by stress and anxiety. In fact, numerous studies have shown that aerobic exercise can be an effective part of treatment for depression and anxiety.

The more you make exercise a habit, the better your mood stays and the lower your stress level, too. But you've got to make a commitment to it. Researchers in Australia studied three groups of people: long-term exercisers, short-term exercisers, and nonexercisers. The long-term exercisers had a more positive outlook on life and were less stressed-out than those in the other two groups, based on the results of questionnaires filled out by the participants.

A consistent exercise program has numerous other benefits to help fortify you against stress. Exercise, for example, improves your mental performance, produces a feeling of well-being, helps control your weight, and reinforces a positive self-image and outlook on life.

Talk it out. Sometimes resolving stress may require more serious measures—like seeing a counselor. A counselor won't solve your problems, but he or she may help you identify strategies to cope with stress and ultimately resolve the underlying issues perpetuating the stress.

Or you may just want to pour your heart out to a friend. Just talking to someone you trust can make you feel much better.

Rearrange your life. Most people have too much on their plates—not food, but activities and commitments. Before long it all spills over into one big mess, and life feels like it's spinning out of control. If that's happening to you, take a look at your life, and based on your priorities, see what you can remove from the plate.

Get some perspective. Sometimes we catastrophize our thinking, turning the proverbial molehill into a mountain. Or we worry about situations over which we have no control. Both mental approaches to life are immobilizing—and unhealthy. They make the stress worse than it really is.

The next time you find yourself mired in this type of thinking, ask yourself: What is the worst thing that can happen? How likely is that to occur? How much difference will this situation make in my life a year from now? Am I likely to even remember it? This type of self-peptalk puts a more positive spin on the situation.

Have fun. To paraphrase an old saying: "All work and no play make Jack a stressed-out boy." Research shows that people who pursue recreational activities on a regular basis in their lives are more satisfied with their lives, and in better health. If you're not having enough fun, sit down and list some fun activities you can integrate into your life—swimming, walking in the park, playing a sport for fun, taking weekend trips, reading more novels, and so forth. Then do them!

A related issue is laughter. Laughter is truly one of the best medicines—and a terrific stress reliever. Like exercise and massage, it also releases endorphins, and these act as muscle relaxants and mood elevators. If nothing seems funny right now, maybe its time to rent a comedy video, go to a comedy club, or read a humorous book.

Get enough rest.   If you're an emotional basket case, take it easy by getting more rest. Rest lets your body renew itself. During this renewal, the body can heal injuries and infections, eliminate toxins and waste products, dissipate stress, replenish fuel stores in the muscle fibers and bloodstream, and restore energy. Rest also allows your immune system to recharge so that you're better protected from disease.

Nurture your soul.   You are more than a body, more than a chemical soup of hormones, and certainly more than a jumble of stresses and problems. For total well-being, plug into spiritual resources such as prayer and meditation. Both do wonders for physical, emotional, and spiritual wellness. Plus, there is a documented scientific link between faith and mental health. People who are religious or come from a religious family have a lower risk of suicide, mental health, drug abuse, alcoholism, and depression.

CHAPTER 7

Easing Anxiety

If you're like most people, you've felt uptight from time to time . . . the butterflies before a big business presentation . . . the stress of an impending deadline . . . worry over mounting bills. While almost everyone feels anxious at one time or another, roughly eighteen million Americans suffer from anxiety so severe and seemingly permanent that it interferes with their daily lives. This type of anxiety is the most common mental health problem in the United States today.

People with severe forms of anxiety are routinely treated with prescription medications. And in most cases, that's as it should be. However, some medicines used to treat anxiety can be highly addictive.

But is there a better way? Could a natural remedy like kava provide relief?

Quite probably—and the results of several well-designed studies bear this out. Conducted over the past ten years, this research demonstrates that people suffering from various types of anxiety improve significantly while supplementing with kava. For treating many mental disorders, kava has joined a growing list of herbal remedies proven to be safe and effective when taken in moderate dosages for short periods of time.

To see where kava might fit in, it helps to understand the various types of anxiety disorders that afflict people.

GENERALIZED ANXIETY DISORDER

If you experience continual but irrational fears that something bad is going to happen—and these feelings persist for six months or longer—you may be suffering from "generalized anxiety disorder." The disorder is particularly serious if it interferes with your ability to carry on day-to-day living. About 8 percent of the population suffers from generalized anxiety disorder, and it affects as many men as women.

The symptoms of generalized anxiety disorder are both emotional and physical. Emotionally, you may feel upset, apprehensive, depressed, irritable, or uneasy, and you may have trouble concentrating on the normal tasks at hand. Your body may react to the anxiety on a physical level with symptoms such as a galloping pulse, clammy skin, shortness of breath, muscular tension, tremors, nausea, light-headedness, insomnia, and fatigue.

What causes generalized anxiety disorder? Like many diseases, there are multiple factors. Research into the innerworkings of the brain has revealed that people suffering from generalized anxiety disorder may have an imbalance of an important brain chemical called GABA, which blocks the transmission of anxiety messages. When treated with drugs that increase GABA activity, anxiety tends to simmer down.

Besides physiological imbalances, deep-seated emotional problems may be at the root of a generalized anxiety disorder. For example, you may have chronic low self-esteem, or a tendency to look at the world in a negative way. Unresolved problems such as an abusive marriage, loss of a loved one, or constant money woes can trigger generalized anxiety disorder, too. Psychiatric counseling and/or a major life change may quell the anxiety.

PANIC DISORDERS

Suddenly, without warning and for no apparent reason, you are gripped with intense terror. You literally freeze, unable to move. Within minutes, your heart starts racing, you're gasping for breath, your chest squeezes in pain, you're shaking and sweating. You feel like you're going to die or go crazy. Then, as quickly as these horrible feelings came on, they leave—until the next episode catches you unawares.

Though symptoms vary from individual to individual, this scenario is all too typical of a "panic attack," a very real and frightening psychological event that characterizes panic disorder. It may last anywhere from ten minutes to a half hour. Nearly three million Americans suffer from this debilitating problem.

At the root of panic disorder may be a chemical imbalance in the brain. As I noted in chapter 6, research has shown that people suffering from panic disorder have an overactive amygdala, the portion of the brain that controls such emotions as fear and anxiety. As revealed by sophisticated brain scans, blood flow and oxygen to this part of the brain are higher than in patients who don't panic. Or panic disorder may have a genetic link, since it tends to run in families. Also, a panic attack may be a symptom of an underlying disease. In fact, more than forty diseases can trigger paniclike reactions.

Panic disorder is typically treated with prescription

mood medications and psychotherapy. A recent study conducted in Germany found exercise to be therapeutic as well. Forty-six patients suffering from moderate to severe panic disorder were randomly assigned to a ten-week treatment program of regular aerobic exercise (running), clomipramine (Anafranil, 112.5 milligrams daily), or placebo pills. (Clomipramine is an antidepressant commonly used to treat people suffering from obsessions and compulsions.) As it turned out, exercise improved anxiety symptoms greatly. When combined with the medication, exercise worked even more effectively.

PHOBIAS

Few of us like to see a snake slither across our path, and who doesn't clutch the armrest when an airplane flight gets turbulent? Natural fears like these are common, but if they become so intense that you won't walk in your garden or board an airplane, you may be suffering from a phobia.

"Phobia" comes from a Greek word meaning "fear" or "flight." Basically, a phobia is a persistent, irrational fear of a place, a situation, or an object. There are literally hundreds of different kinds of phobias. Fear of speaking in front of an audience, for example, is a common phobia. A more serious phobia is agoraphobia, in which a person is afraid of being trapped in a public place, unable to escape. Consequently, the agoraphobic stays home rather than risk the possible terror. Panic disorder sufferers often become agoraphobic because they fear being seized by a panic attack while in public. Nearly a million people, most of them women, suffer from agoraphobia.

Unless a phobia interferes with daily living, there's no cause for concern. But if a phobia keeps you from living a normal life, it should be diagnosed and treated. Phobias can be successfully overcome with a combination of medication, counseling, and gradual exposure to the fear-evoking situation.

OBSESSIVE-COMPULSIVE DISORDER

If you saw the hit movie *As Good As It Gets* starring Jack Nicholson as an obsessive-compulsive writer, you have a pretty good picture of what this disorder is all about. In essence, people who suffer from this disorder exhibit compulsions—rituals they must perform before they can begin another activity. Examples of ritualistic behavior include: repetitive hand-washing, excessive neatness, checking and rechecking to make sure something isn't forgotten, or performing an activity in a series of senseless steps. If the rituals can't be completed as desired, the sufferer may feel an overwhelming sense of anxiety or despair.

Obsessions may involve the mind as well. The obsessive-compulsive may be plagued with persistent thoughts of violence or sex or fears of becoming infected with germs.

No one really knows what produces this disorder, although research points to a physiological cause. It is treatable with medication and behavioral therapy, however.

POST-TRAUMATIC STRESS DISORDER

What was once called shell shock or battle fatigue is now known as post-traumatic stress disorder, or PTSD, because it is not limited to soldiers harmed by war. Any trauma beyond the range of normal human experience—rape, tornado, bombing, automobile accident, airplane crash, and so forth—can induce this disorder in survivors of the trauma. Even so, veterans are its main victims, with as many as 800,000 Vietnam vets suffering from PTSD.

Symptoms of PTSD include flashbacks of the trauma, hallucinations, estrangement from others, a sense of hopelessness, insomnia, and extreme anxiety or panic. These may surface immediately after the trauma, or be delayed by six months or longer. Seemingly benign incidents or associations can spark a PTSD attack—a loud noise, a certain odor, even a locale—and the horror of the trauma comes back, unbidden, in torrents of panic.

Scientists now theorize that the amygdala may be involved in generating the PTSD panic response. Normally the amygdala helps us react appropriately to threatening situations. But in PTSD sufferers, those reactions can go haywire. That's because the amygdala somehow pairs innocuous environmental cues (like a noise or a smell) with a traumatic memory, triggering a pathological reliving of the terror.

Other research suggests that trauma may harm the hippocampus. Two studies have found that people with trauma histories have smaller hippocampi than normal.

Trauma survivors also have abnormally low levels of stress hormones such as cortisol. Research has also found that trauma damages certain receptors in the brain and reduces their number. Consequently, these receptors can't properly regulate the amount of adrenaline that's released. There's too much of a surge, which tends to set off flashbacks.

Although tranquilizers can reduce the symptoms, no drug has yet been found to truly conquer the intense fear and anxiety of a PTSD episode. What is needed is some way to alter the biochemistry of the amygdala, and thus block the fear. Since kava is known to act on the amygdala, the herb may prove of some use in treating PTSD, but this is only speculation.

KAVA AND ANXIETY

People continue to ask me about kava: Is there really science behind this stuff? You bet—and plenty of it.

One of the earliest—and most fascinating—studies on kava and anxiety was conducted in the late 1980s. Scientists at the University of Vienna explored the effect of kava (specifically, kavain) on the brain waves of fifteen psychologically and physically healthy volunteers. The measurement of brain waves provided important clues to kava's benefit. When you're anxious, or very stressed-out, brain waves called "beta waves" go haywire. By contrast, when you're relaxed, or in a meditative state, brain waves called "alpha waves" are more active.

Ideally, to curb anxiety, you want to reduce beta activity and increase alpha activity. Interestingly, at 200-milligram doses of kavain, alpha activity increased, while beta activity dropped off—an indication that kavain helped reduce anxiety and calm the body.

KAVA AXES ANXIETY WITHIN ONE WEEK

In a 1991 study, fifty-eight patients suffering from anxiety of nonmental origin were divided into two groups—a kava group, which took a kava extract (100 milligrams three times daily), and a placebo group. The experiment lasted four weeks, and after weeks one, two, and four of treatment, the subjects were assessed using a reputable test to evaluate anxiety. Kava's action was surprisingly rapid. In just one week, those who took kava supplements showed a significant reduction in anxiety symptoms and were dramatically better by the end of the study. (Those in the placebo group didn't fare as well.) No one reported experiencing a single side effect, either.

KAVA BANISHES MENOPAUSE-PRODUCED ANXIETY

If there were a supplement you could pop to cut the tension, or modulate the mood swings that go along with menopause, wouldn't you want it in your medicine chest? Absolutely—and kava is that supplement. In a 1991 study of women (ages forty-five to fifty) experiencing anxiety and depression associated with menopause, twenty were treated with a kava extract standardized to 70 percent kavalactones, and twenty with a placebo, for eight weeks. Treatment success was measured using a variety of standardized tests. Those taking kava improved significantly, with a 58 percent reduction in symptoms, and experienced much improved mood states, while those on the placebo showed little or no improvement. Overall, the women undergoing kava therapy simply felt better than before.

KAVA TAMES THE TENSION

The largest, most carefully controlled study of kava's antianxiety effects was conducted at Jena University in 1997. Researchers there recruited 101 outpatients who were suffering from anxiety, obsessive-compulsive disorder, or phobias. These people were given either 100 milligrams of kava three times a day (the formulation was a special extract containing 70 percent kavalactones, and available commercially in Germany), or a placebo. Several psychological tests to assess anxiety and mood were administered, and the study lasted twenty-five weeks.

Eight weeks into the study, those taking kava showed significant alleviation of their symptoms, compared to those on the placebo. As the study progressed, they began to feel even better! And by the end of the study, the researchers rated the kava group as "very much improved," while the placebo group showed much less improvement. Plus, there were virtually no reported side effects. The researchers noted, too, that their results support the use of kava as a treatment alternative to the antidepressants and tranquilizers typically used to treat anxiety.

Taken together, these studies show that kava is remarkable in its ability to treat anxiety—and to do so virtually without side effects. As research into kava's antianxiety benefits continues, we may see kava become an important line of defense against this troubling mood disorder.

SOME RESOURCES

Need more information about anxiety? Here's a list of resources to help you:

- National Institute of Mental Health information line, 1–888–8–ANXIETY.
- Anxiety Disorders Association of America, 11900 Parklawn Dr. Suite 100, Rockville, MD 20852. 301–231–9350.
- American Psychiatric Association, 1400 K Street NW, Washington, DC 20005. 202–682–6000.
- American Psychological Association, 750 1st Street NE, Washington, DC 20002–4242. 202–336–5500.
- National Mental Health Association, 1021 Prince Street, Alexandria, VA 22314–2971. 1–800–969–6642.

CHAPTER 8

Beating the Blues

Sadness. Despair. A sense that life's not worth living. These are just a few signs of "depression," a mental illness that affects one of every four Americans. Depression is a very common mental disorder—in fact, it has been dubbed "the common cold" of psychiatric problems—but it is the most treatable, provided the sufferer seeks treatment.

Getting treatment is vital, not only to restore mental health but also to prevent some serious health problems. Depression is a risk factor for heart disease. It increases the risk for broken bones. And it compromises immunity against disease. Tragically 15 percent of all depressed people kill themselves, according to studies. Two thirds of these visit a physician in the month immediately prior to the suicide.

Where does kava fit in? It is speculated that one cause of depression may be an overstimulated amygdala—the region of the brain that involves emotion. Kavalactones appear to work on the amygdala—so do certain drugs—

and thus may help alleviate some forms of mild depression.

From a down-in-the-dumps mood to suicidal tendencies, depression is a complex problem, with a wide range of symptoms, including withdrawal, inactivity, loss of appetite, feelings of helplessness, and mental anguish. There are several classifications of depression, but for the sake of simplicity, I shall group them into two: situational depression and biochemical depression.

SITUATIONAL DEPRESSION

You lose your job . . . your spouse leaves you . . . a loved one becomes ill. Distressing life experiences like these can trigger a protracted episode of the blues, known technically as situational depression. Its symptoms include:

- a sense of hopelessness
- grief
- shattered self-esteem
- anxiety or worry
- irritability
- a retreat from social relationships

Situational depression is often a side effect of certain life choices, too. Alcohol, for example, acts as a depressant, although it may temporarily boost your mood. It also interferes with the dreaming periods of sleep, known as rapid-eye-movement (REM) sleep. This leads to fatigue and, with it, depression.

Prolonged dieting triggers depression, too, particularly if you do not eat enough carbohydrate-rich foods. Carbohydrate supplies glucose, the principal brain fuel. Deprived of enough glucose, the brain cannot adequately make serotonin, a brain chemical associated with mood. Hence, you may feel anxious, tense, and depressed while following a low-carbohydrate diet. Eating enough carbohydrates such as breads, cereals, potatoes, or pasta reverses these feelings.

Normally situational depression resolves itself as the disappointment or loss fades and you begin to get on with your life. Yet if the depression persists without resolution, you may need counseling to explore solutions to life problems, resolve feelings of hopelessness or low self-esteem, or overcome self-defeating ways of thinking.

Many depressed people reach for one of the commonly prescribed drugs for depression. However, natural agents may provide a healthier, more workable solution as part of therapy, and one of these is kava. It works best against situational depression by elevating your mood, soothing tension, and helping you cope. The herb exerts its mood-boosting action by positively altering brain chemistry and relaxing your muscles. Clinical trials show that kava most definitely increases your sense of well-being and lifts you out of the dumps.

It is well-established medically that stressful events in your life can trigger depression. Since kava helps you temporarily cope with stress, it could potentially lessen the likelihood that your stress will turn to depression, or it could head depression off at the pass.

In its feature on kava aired in June 1998, ABC's 20/20 recounted the compelling story of a woman whose husband, a decorated marine pilot, had died accidentally. After the shock wore off, grief set in—and with it, all the life-weary burdens of coping alone. She wanted something to get her through the grieving, but did not want to go on drugs. A psychiatrist recommended that she take 60 milligrams of kavalactones three times a day. And it made a huge difference. She felt like she could cope, be strong, and get through the painful, often immobilizing period of grief.

If you're in the grip of a painful time and just need a way to cope, talk to your psychiatrist or physician about taking kava. It may be just the temporary strategy you need to improve your mood and return to normal well-being.

BIOCHEMICAL DEPRESSION

A person stricken with biochemical depression experiences desperate feelings that go beyond a mere "bad funk" or just being in the doldrums. Biochemical depression is a perplexing and very serious psychiatric illness that affects both mind and body.

Its origins lie in the brain. Governing behavior is a regular ebb and flow of brain chemicals (hormones) known as neurotransmitters. They transmit messages by spewing out from the tail end of one nerve cell into another nerve cell across a "synapse" (the tiny space between nerve cells). It is thought that one of the chief causes of biochemical depression is low levels of the neurotransmitters serotonin and norepinephrine in these synapses. When there is an imbalance or short supply of neurotransmitters at this passageway, the result can spell trouble.

Biochemical depression (also termed clinical depression) manifests itself in the following symptoms:

- low energy and feelings of exhaustion
- persistent sadness
- anxiety and tension
- insomnia
- loss of interest in pleasurable activities, including sex

- memory problems, forgetfulness, poor concentration
- irritability and crankiness with little or no provocation
- unhappiness
- lack of self-esteem
- appetite problems, either loss of appetite or binge eating
- physical problems that do not respond to treatment, including headaches, digestive disorders, joint pain, and chronic respiratory infections
- mood swings
- thoughts of suicide

Under the broad classification of biochemical depression are some subcategories. Manic-depressive illness, also called "bipolar disorder," is characterized by alternating patterns of emotional highs and lows. There is also unipolar depression, often termed "clinical depression." It lacks the emotional highs seen in bipolar depression.

Millions of Americans also suffer from seasonal affective disorder (SAD), another form of biochemical depression. Sufferers get severely depressed in the winter, experience headaches, get irritable, and have frequent crying spells. This extreme form of the "winter blahs" may be linked to the body's biological clock, which is involved in regulating hormones, and hence, mood. SAD sufferers respond to light therapy, because it may stimulate the activity of neurotransmitters, particularly serotonin. Scientists think that certain parts of the brain are stimulated by sunlight.

A milder form of biochemical depression can occur premenstrually. More than one hundred symptoms have been identified in women suffering from "PMS," or premenstrual syndrome. Among the most common are depression, irritability, and anxiety. The physiological causes of PMS have been hotly debated in scientific circles, but now many medical researchers agree that at its root are neurotransmitter abnormalities. The most often blamed neurotransmitter is the mood-lifting serotonin. Low levels of serotonin may cause mild depression. Thus, physicians often treat severe PMS-related depression with antidepressants known to restore serotonin balance.

There's exciting new proof that kava can treat PMS-related depression, too—and do so without the worrisome side effects of some antidepressants. In the breakthrough study described in the previous chapter, researchers in Germany showed for the first time that taking 100 milligrams of a kava extract three times a day is a bona fide remedy for premenstrual depression. In this double-blind, placebo-controlled study of forty women, half the group got kava and half got a placebo for a period of eight weeks. Prior to the study, their symptoms were assessed with standardized tests, and during the study, the women kept diaries of how they felt.

The result: Kava lifted depression, imparted a sense of well-being, and reduced the severity of PMS symptoms significantly. In fact, the women taking kava began to feel better in just one week. Best of all, the kava-takers experienced no side effects.

Of course, much more research is needed on kava and depression. Researchers have barely scratched the surface, but its therapeutic promise is thrilling nonetheless.

Another excellent natural antidepressant is the herb St. John's wort, proven over and over again in scientific studies to reduce and reverse depression. Amazingly, St. John's wort is currently the only agent that is effective on serotonin *and* norepinephrine. (Prozac and other synthetic antidepressants work only on single brain chemicals.)

Further, St. John's wort may positively influence dopamine, another neurotransmitter involved in mood.

What's more, an average monthly supply of St. John's wort costs about twenty dollars—less than a tenth of Prozac, one of the main prescription remedies for depression. A supply of Prozac costs one hundred to two hundred dollars a month.

(For more information on the remarkable benefits of St. John's wort, see chapter 12.)

TREATING AND DEFEATING DEPRESSION

Because of chemical imbalances in the brain, some people may need to be on prescription medication for life. But not all patients fully respond to medication alone. Depression can be such a complex disease that it typically requires a more comprehensive approach.

If your depression is nonchemical or of a situational nature, counseling and lifestyle changes may be in order. While medication—including kava—may help you temporarily, you should not lean on these agents forever. What follows is a look at various nondrug approaches that as part of a comprehensive treatment approach are effective in treating depression:

Seek psychiatric counseling. Counseling can help you identify why your depression exists and give you constructive guidelines for resolving it. Also, try a type of counseling called "cognitive therapy." You'll learn how to slip out of self-defeating thought patterns and think more positively and realistically about the world around you.

Get moving. In addition to counseling, exercise is emerging as an important adjunct to treatment. One reason is that it releases natural mood-elevating chemicals called endorphins. In one study, thirty to forty minutes of walking and running three times a week compared favorably with psychotherapy in the treatment of eight depressed patients. Six of the patients were diagnosed as "essentially well" after three weeks of exercise therapy, and they stayed that way for one year afterward.

Another study examined the responses of forty-three depressed women to either aerobic exercise (dancing, jogging, and running), relaxation exercise, or nonexercise. The women who exercised aerobically experienced significantly greater decreases in depression than did all the other participants. The researchers concluded that "participation in a program of strenuous aerobic exercise was effective for reducing depression."

Modify your environment. Moods can worsen if you're lonely or isolated—or in surroundings or around people that "bring you down." You may have to change your lifestyle, or make new social contacts. Volunteering is a good way to reduce social isolation and meet new people. Pick a cause you want to support, and volunteer your time and talents to help make a difference. You won't be sorry, and you'll be better off, physically and mentally.

Research shows you can experience the same physiological changes when you help others as you do when you exercise. Heart rate and breathing decrease, and feel-good endorphins are released—all of which power up your immune system. This is the exact opposite of what happens when you're depressed. Other studies show that people who regularly volunteer their time to worthy causes are less likely to get depressed.

Be creative. Tap in to your talents, whether it's painting a picture, tending a garden, or writing a poem. Creative pursuits will give you a sense of accomplishment, in addition to rescuing you from the doldrums.

Join a support group. Meeting with other people who share your problem can be an effective form of therapy, especially when combined with individual counseling. Sharing with others helps address underlying problems contributing to depression and helps you see that you're not alone in your struggle. Check with your local hospital or mental health center to see if such groups meet in your community.

Nourish your body. A number of vitamin and mineral deficiencies have been linked to symptoms of depression. Deficiencies of iron, thiamine, selenium, magnesium, and carbohydrates, for example, produce depressive symptoms, low moods, anxiety, and fatigue. A balanced diet may do wonders. Also, eat fatty fish a few times a week. Salmon, tuna, herring, and mackerel are full of omega-3 fatty acids. One type of omega-3 is DHA, which makes up 30 percent of certain brain cell membranes. Studies have found that levels of omega-3s (including DHA) are lower in patients with depression. You might be able to partially protect yourself against depression by including more fish in your diet. (For information on other nutrients that affect mood, see chapter 13.)

Get a checkup. As well, be sure to have a complete medical checkup if you are suffering from depression. There are many conditions that produce depressive symptoms, including thyroid malfunctions, menopause, diabetes, and anemia.

CHAPTER 9

Overcoming Insomnia

Is sound sleep only a dream? If so, you're not alone. Health experts now affirm that insomnia, which means too little sleep, has become one of the most pervasive health problems in the United States, responsible for personality disorders, traffic accidents, debilitating fatigue, memory loss, poor physical performance, and illness. As many as 60 percent of us have trouble getting enough shut-eye, at least occasionally. Additionally, insomnia is the third most common complaint heard by doctors, after colds and headaches.

Yet sleep is an absolutely vital component of health. If we don't get enough, we're shortchanging our bodies of valuable, health-promoting rest. In fact, slumbering seven to eight hours nightly is one of the chief health habits shared by people who stay fit well into their golden years.

Insomnia takes different forms. You may experience temporary sleeplessness due to minor stress or worry. Or you may have trouble falling asleep. There is also the type of insomnia that may awaken you frequently during the night, or make you wake up too early.

Each type of insomnia can last for a couple of weeks, or
become chronic and long-term. If you have difficulty falling asleep every night, or most nights, for a month or
longer, you probably have chronic insomnia. However, any
degree of insomnia can damage your health by weakening
your immune system and making you more susceptible to
illness. When you do not get enough sleep, you're less
alert, de-energized, and certainly more prone to illness.

WHAT'S KEEPING YOU UP AT NIGHT?

Insomnia is caused by a number of medical, emotional, or
behavioral factors, including:

Hormonal changes preceding menopause. Women having hot
flashes at night, termed "night sweats," are often kept
awake by these sensations and do not get enough restorative sleep as a result.

Anxiety, stress, or tension. In a survey conducted by the National Sleep Foundation, most people said job stress and
other worries kept them sleepless most nights. Psychological problems are frequently at the root of sleep disturbances. Anxiety, stress, and tension, in particular, are the
most common causes of insomnia and often require treatment by a qualified therapist, particularly if the anxiety-
producing situations are difficult to resolve.

Depression. Although there are various types of depression,
they often share the same symptoms. One of these is
disturbed sleep. Depression is a complex disorder that
usually requires professional treatment.

Physical pain. Countless illnesses, injuries, and other medical conditions produce pain, some of it chronic. It is very

difficult to sleep, or stay asleep, when your body hurts. Taken at night, pain-relieving medications offer some comfort.

Hypoglycemia (low blood sugar). Often requiring dietary and medical management, hypoglycemia is a condition in which concentrations of blood sugar (glucose) are below normal. When blood sugar is in short supply, the brain (which is fueled by glucose) and other body cells become starved for energy. In response, the body starts producing brain chemicals that stimulate the release of blood sugar. This rise in blood sugar can wake you up if it occurs during your normal sleep hours. If you think you suffer from hypoglycemia, have your doctor test you for it.

Caffeine. Drinking excessive amounts of coffee, tea, or cola beverages can keep you awake nights because they contain caffeine, a known stimulant.

Alcohol and drugs. Although alcohol is relaxing and makes you feel sleepy, it actually interferes with normal sleep patterns. Also, the use of certain medications may actively hinder sleep. Talk to your physician or pharmacist if you suspect that a medication is keeping you up nights.

If you're suffering from chronic insomnia, the root of your problem may not be so easily identified. In 30 percent of people diagnosed with chronic insomnia, no cause can be pinpointed.

SNOOZE AND LOSE: THE TROUBLE WITH SLEEPING PILLS

If a medical basis for your insomnia has been ruled out, your doctor may prescribe sleeping pills. Each year, about

25 percent of all adult Americans take some kind of prescription medication for insomnia. The most often prescribed sleep aids are a class of drugs known as the benzodiazepines. Among the benzodiazepines prescribed specifically for insomnia include temazepam (Restoril), estazolam (Prosom), quazepam (Doral), flurazepam (Dalmane), and trizolam (Halcion). All of these are potentially addictive. Over time, your body becomes accustomed to the dosage, until you require greater amounts of the drug to fall asleep. According to *The PDR Family Guide to Prescription Drugs*, dependence may occur with these medications if not taken exactly as prescribed. (For more information on benzodiazepines, see Chapter 11.)

Ironically, some sleeping pills may interfere with normal sleep cycles, particularly if you abruptly discontinue the medication. Withdrawing from the drugs may cause a "rebound" in sleeplessness, meaning that insomnia often gets worse. According to *The PDR Family Guide to Prescription Drugs*, some sleeping pills have potential side effects that include dizziness and drowsiness. You should check with your physician or pharmacist for information on other possible side effects.

Also, there are now some newer sleeping pills with fewer potential side effects. These belong to a class of medications known as nonbenzodiazepines. (For more information on these, see Chapter 11.)

If pain from an illness is keeping you awake at night, sleeping pills may be appropriate.

Another course of action is to try over-the-counter medications such as antihistamines, which are usually found in cold, allergy, and sinus products. Antihistamines induce drowsiness and sleep, but leave you in a fog of fatigue upon rising. As with benzodiazepines, your body can adapt to them. Antihistamines have side effects, too, like constipation, dry mouth, and visual problems.

So what's a tired body to do? Increasingly, more people are turning to natural sleep remedies, particularly herbs such as kava. In Germany and other European countries, kava is approved as a treatment for insomnia.

Kava works by alleviating the stress and anxiety that are perpetuating the insomnia. As a natural sedative and nightcap, kava acts on brain areas that regulate sleep. Plus, best of all, you'll wake up feeling refreshed—without groggy aftereffects.

To understand how kava works to overcome insomnia, it's important to know what happens to your body and brain while you're asleep. By measuring brain waves with high-tech equipment, scientists have discovered that a person goes through different stages of sleep during slumber. You move from wakefulness to drowsiness to moderate sleep to deep restorative sleep.

Deep restorative sleep is known as rapid-eye-movement (REM) sleep. During REM, your eyes dart around rapidly as you dream. Not only do your eyes move, but your heart rate, breathing, and the blood flow to your brain also increase. Your brain waves are very active during REM sleep, as are your eye movements; but your muscles are quite inactive and virtually paralyzed. This is because your brain transmits signals that relax your muscles so that you won't physically act out your dreams. During sleep you undergo several periods of REM sleep, usually occurring about once every ninety minutes and totaling about one and a half hours.

As each REM period ends, you move into non-REM (or non-dreaming) sleep. Your brain waves become slower, although there are brief bursts of electrical activity from the brain termed "sleep spindles." During non-

REM sleep, brain activity, as recorded by electroencephalographs (EEG), is characterized by "delta" waves, less active signals that are given off when you're awake or in REM sleep.

Scientists speculate that it is during delta-wave sleep that your body repairs itself physically. Thus, if your delta-wave sleep is disturbed, you're likely to feel dragged out and unrefreshed upon waking. REM sleep, on the other hand, is critical for recovering from mental stress. Deprived of REM sleep, you're likely to lose mental focus and alertness.

KAVA AND INSOMNIA: WHAT SCIENCE SAYS

In scientific experiments with animals and humans, kava has been found to naturally promote delta-wave sleep—which is why you feel refreshed, instead of fatigued, after taking kava to help you sleep.

Various sleep experiments have been performed on animals treated with a kava extract. In one study, pigeons given kava slept for ten to twelve hours. And monkeys on kava have fallen asleep within fifteen minutes, then slumbering for as long as fifteen hours. Other animal experiments have combined kava with prescription sleeping pills such as barbiturates, making the barbiturates more effective. Some scientists believe such a combination could be effective in weaning insomniacs off sleeping pills.

In 1991 a German study was published, demonstrating the effectiveness of kava as a healthy sleep aid. Researchers enlisted two sets of six volunteers (three women and nine men, between the ages of twenty and thirty-one). One set of volunteers was given 50 milligrams of a standardized kava extract three times a day; the other set, 100 milligrams, also three times a day. The experiment lasted four days and nights. During that time, the researchers recorded the volunteers' brain waves using an EEG, as well as their muscular activity using an electromyograph (EMG). A number of fascinating findings emerged from the study:

1. Kava elevated EEG sleep-spindle density (it was 20 percent higher in eleven of the twelve volunteers). This indicated that the volunteers sank into a deeper sleep earlier and faster.
2. The periods of deepest sleep were enhanced—without any changes or interruptions in sleep.
3. With the higher dose of kava, volunteers fell asleep faster.
4. Discontinuation of kava produced no rebound effect (as sleeping pills may do if discontinued abruptly).

Kava works very well with other sleep-producing herbs such as valerian, chamomile, passionflower, and hops (these are covered in chapter 12). Also, some supplement makers have combined kava with the naturally occurring brain hormone melatonin, which, like kava, enhances delta-wave sleep.

SLEEP GREAT EVERY NIGHT

To get and stay fit, you must get sound shut-eye. Sleep is as critical to the body as exercise and nutrition because it gives your body time to recover and revive. You know you've had a restful night when you can wake up without your alarm clock and feel refreshed for the rest of the day. If you're having trouble achieving that kind of slumber, here are some practical tips to help you:

1. Eat a nutritious diet. A poor diet can cause an array of physical and emotional problems. Populate your diet with lots of fresh fruits and vegetables, whole grains, lean proteins, and dairy foods.

   Supplement your diet, too. Often we don't get all the nutrients we need. Supplementation with a multivitamin/mineral product offers good nutritional insurance. Also, B-complex vitamins have been shown to help alleviate sleeplessness.

2. Exercise regularly, but moderately. Physical activity helps you slumber. But don't exercise too late in the day, or in the evening, because exercise stimulates the metabolism and builds up natural chemicals in the body. This can have a stimulating effect on your system.

3. Go to bed at a regular time and maintain a regular sleep schedule.

4. Establish calming prebedtime activities. Some ideas: take a hot bath, sip a mug of chamomile tea, have a massage, or read an uplifting book. By contrast, do not watch violent television dramas or horror shows before retiring. These can and do produce nightmares.

5. Darken your room.

6. Keep your room well ventilated.

7. Cut out sleep-robbing substances such as caffeine and alcohol. (Eliminate coffee and caffeine-containing foods after midday.)

8. If you do have to get up at night, don't turn on any lights. Exposure to light in the middle of the night can block your body's production of melatonin, a hormone that regulates your sleep/wake cycle. It could be harder for you to fall asleep again.

9. Make sure your mattress is supportive and comfortable.

10. Create a neat, restful sleep environment.

CHAPTER 10

More Medical Miracles from Kava

Islanders have used kava for a slew of medical problems (see table 2 on page 123)—and for good reason. It does the body a world of good, and its power is only just being discovered by modern medical science. Here's a look at what we know about kava and the promise it holds in treating a host of other medical conditions, from illnesses to addictions to sexual dysfunction.

RELIEVING PAIN

For thousands of years, South Pacific islanders have used kava to make the pain go away. It has worked for them—and it may just work for us, too.

Each year, we spend more than $80 billion to relieve our aches and pains. Those dollars are spent mostly on pain-killing medications termed "analgesics." There are several different types: aspirin, acetaminophen, narcotics, anti-inflammatory drugs such as ibuprofen, tranquilizers, muscle-relaxants, and local anesthetics. The choice of analgesic varies according to the degree of pain, and the type of injury or illness.

Interestingly, kava could be a jack-of-all-trades when it comes to managing pain, since it shares many of the characteristics of the categories of analgesics listed above. Take aspirin and morphine (a narcotic), for example. Kava's two pain-relieving chemicals, dihydrokavain and dihydromethysticin, have analgesic properties nearly twice as potent as aspirin.

Both kavalactones have been compared to morphine, too. But neither is as strong. You'd have to take about fifty times as much dihydrokavain and dihydromethysticin to get the same pain-killing effect as morphine. Still, kava and its active constituents could be effective painkillers.

How kava works to stop pain is a puzzle, though. Scientists know that morphine and other narcotics such as codeine act by blocking certain pain receptors in the brain and nervous system. Does kava do the same? To find out, researchers administered naloxone to mice that had been given various kava extracts (kavain, methysticin, dihydrokavain, and dihydromethysticin). Naloxone is a drug that reverses the effects of morphine and other narcotics and blocks their pain-killing action. If kava worked like morphine, naloxone would reverse its effects, too. But naloxone had no effect. It didn't prevent the kava extracts from stopping pain. This finding led the scientists to conclude that kava does not work on the same areas of the brain and nervous system as morphine does, but kills pain through some other pathway.

Kava also acts like an anti-inflammatory drug—which is probably why Tahitians used it in the 1800s to treat rheumatism. Inflammation is caused by increased blood flow, which in turn produces pain, swelling, redness, and heat. At the injury site, painful agents called prostaglandins are among the inflammatory substances released. Prostaglandins are manufactured by enzymes. Anti-inflammatory drugs such as ibuprofen and naproxen interfere with the action of these enzymes, thus blocking the body's production of prostaglandins and taming the pain. At least one kava experiment has found that kavain does the same thing.

Part of kava's analgesic benefit is also due to its anesthetic action. The herb numbs the mouth much in the same way as Novocain and similar injectable medications. You might try it in extract form to soothe the symptoms of sore gums, canker sores, or toothache. Kava also comes in a spray, which you can squirt toward the back of your mouth to ease the pain of a sore throat.

Four kavalactones have been identified as potent anesthetics: kavain, dihydrokavain, methysticin, and dihydromethysticin. Animal experiments have documented that all four are as strong as cocaine when applied topically! In animal studies, dihydromethysticin, in particular, has been shown to intensify and extend the anesthetic action of barbiturates, which are sometimes given to patients prior to surgery. The clinical significance of these findings isn't clear, but down the road this could mean the use of smaller doses of barbiturates for surgery. A red flag though: Don't take kava if you're about to undergo surgery. Combined with anesthesia, kava could be dangerous.

Kava may be effective for people suffering from fibromyalgia, a rather mysterious ailment characterized by aches, pain, and stiffness in the joints and muscles. It is usually treated with anti-inflammatory drugs, relaxation techniques, massages, and regular exercise. Because kava is an excellent muscle relaxant, it relaxes the often painful muscle spasms that accompany this disease.

Painful menstrual cramping might be eased by kava, too. Mild abdominal cramps are fairly normal on the first day or two of your period. But for 10 percent of menstruating women, the pain is so severe that they cannot function unless taking painkillers. Cramping is most likely caused by excessive levels of prostaglandins. These chemicals cause the uterus to contract, and painful cramping results. But since kava is known to relax the uterus, it may be helpful in relieving cramps and pain—but usually without the side effects of prescription painkillers.

TREATING URINARY TRACT INFECTIONS (UTIs)

Urine is a sea of fluids, salt, and waste products. Bacteria may be present, and normally the body can rid itself of microorganisms through the process of urination. But when it can't, urinary tract infections (UTIs) set in. UTIs can be caused by sexual activity, blockages, hormonal changes, and poor immunity, among other things. There are numerous symptoms; one of the most painful is a burning sensation when you urinate. The pain can be relieved by kava because kava acts like an anesthetic, producing a dulling effect. However, kava won't get rid of the actual infection.

CONTROLLING SEIZURES

A small body of evidence shows that kava is an "anticonvulsive," meaning that it prevents seizures. A seizure is an uncontrolled spread of electrical activity in the brain that may cause changes in physical motion and behavior. Although seizure is most associated with epilepsy, many seizures are caused by trauma, disease, tumors, infections, or drug reactions.

There are various types of seizures. The two most common are the grand mal and petit mal. In a grand mal seizure, you lose consciousness, your muscles contract and stiffen, and a series of convulsions follows. Eventually the convulsions slow down, and the seizure ends, sometimes with a few minutes of sleep before consciousness returns. Usually there is no memory of the seizure, although the person may emerge from it feeling confused.

In the petit mal seizure, many small seizures may occur throughout a day, though each one usually lasts only a few seconds. There may be some chewing motion, fluttering of the eyelids, mild twitching of the head and arms, staring into space, or no movement at all. Recovery takes just a few seconds, and there is usually no recollection that the seizure has occurred.

Medication controls or greatly reduces seizures in the majority of people who are affected. Among the most commonly prescribed medications are carbamazephine (Tegretol), clonazepam (Klonopin), phenytoin (Dilantin), phenobarbital, and valproic acid (Depakene or Depakote). These drugs have various side effects, according to *The PDR Family Guide to Prescription Drugs.* You should check with your physician and pharmacist for a list of possible side effects associated with each medication.

In light of this, could there be a better way to treat seizures?

Possibly, but not conclusively. In laboratory studies, animals pretreated with kavalactones survived when given lethal injections of strychnine, known to produce violent muscular contractions similar to what an epileptic has in a grand mal seizure.

In the 1960s an experiment was conducted in the

United States to find out whether kava could help control epileptic seizures. Nine prison inmates were treated with either 6 grams of pure kava root or 1 gram of its alcoholic extract. Both treatments did indeed help control seizures, but after several weeks, the prisoners started experiencing side effects such as skin yellowing. As a result the researchers began treating the inmates with 1200 milligrams per day of dihydromethysticin, one of kava's active constituents. It helped reduce the number of grand mal seizures but had no effect on petit mal seizures. The experiment was stopped because the high doses of dihydromethysticin caused swelling and redness around the eyes, as well as diarrhea and vomiting.

More recently, a study published in 1996 found that kavain suppressed the release of glutamate, one of the many chemicals that transmit messages in the brain. Glutamate is a major "excitatory" neurotransmitter—that is, it causes brain cells to keep firing rather than to stop firing. But sometimes glutamate goes haywire and overstimulates brain cells. Areas of the brain become overexcited, causing seizures and other types of neurological disorders. The data suggest that by suppressing glutamate, kavain could theoretically calm overexcited areas of the brain and possibly quell seizures. Clearly though, more research is needed to substantiate kava's therapeutic use in treating seizures.

TREATING STROKE

Without question, the computerlike brain is the most intricate and fascinating organ in the human body, yet it is still vulnerable to various illnesses and accidents. One of these is stroke, a disturbance to the brain's blood supply. The National Stroke Association defines stroke as "a sudden, usually severe impairment of body functions caused by a disruption in the supply of blood to the brain." Each year, approximately 400,000 to 600,000 Americans suffer a stroke, and nearly 150,000 people die from this condition. It is the third leading cause of death and the leading cause of disability among adults.

The brain uses more oxygen and nutrients than any other part of the body, all fed to the brain by the body's network of blood vessels. If an artery supply to the brain ruptures, bleeds, or becomes clogged, a stroke is the result. A disturbance like this lasting more than a few seconds can kill brain cells because they become starved for oxygen. Medically, a lack of blood flow to tissue (including brain tissue) is called ischemia.

In one laboratory study, researchers pretreated rats and mice with a kava extract or individual kava constituents, then induced ischemia to the rodents' brains. What they found was intriguing: The kava constituents methysticin and dihydromethysticin appeared to protect the brain from ischemia. In other words, fewer brain cells died off. Of course, this is just one study—done with animals only—so it's too early to tell whether kava could have any real benefit in treating stroke patients or helping them survive.

HEALTHY BLOOD CLOTTING

The kava constituent, kavain, may affect the way your blood clots. When you bleed after a cut or injury to a blood vessel, blood cells called platelets rush to the injury site. There, they form a sticky clump, or clot, that closes off the opening in the blood vessel. Under normal circumstances such as this, clotting keeps you from bleeding to death.

A fatty acid in the blood called arachidonic acid assists platelets in clumping together. But too much of this fat can cause abnormal clotting to occur. (Heart attacks are caused by dangerous blood clots that block arteries, choking off blood flow to the heart.)

In test tubes, researchers pretreated human platelets with kavain, then added arachidonic acid to the same platelets to induce clumping. But no clumping occurred. Kavain demonstrated an anticlotting effect.

Aspirin decreases clotting, too. That's why many cardiologists recommend an aspirin-a-day regimen to their heart patients. But as yet, no one has compared which agent is the stronger anticoagulant. What's more, it is too early to tell whether kavain should be taken, as aspirin is, by people at risk for heart attack.

EASING THE ANXIETY OF CANCER

The understandable emotional distress of a cancer diagnosis and subsequent treatment can often thwart the recovery process. As I explained in chapter 7, stress can harm your immune system. But when you calm the stress, your immune system is in a better position to do its job—protecting and healing your body. A few health care institutions around the country are tapping into the healing power of herbs to ease the stress of patients with cancer and other life-threatening illnesses. Kava is among the herbs with the potential to ease anxiety, depression, insomnia, and other emotional symptoms that accompany cancer. Other herbs with antianxiety power include chamomile and valerian. (For more information on these herbs, see chapter 12.)

KICKING THE HABIT

Each year, smoking kills approximately 400,000 Americans—more than died in World War II and Vietnam combined. Lung cancer, chronic lung disease, heart attacks—these are the chief smoking-related diseases that claim human life. Yet death from smoking doesn't have to happen. It is the single largest preventable cause of premature death and disability.

Nicotine, the drug in tobacco, is one of the most addictive substances on earth. Its powerful hold on the body makes smoking one of the toughest habits to kick. While there is no one tried-and-true method for quitting smoking, the decision to quit generally begins with the commitment of the smoker. Other supportive aids such as nicotine gum and a change in routine may help, too.

Many people find that smoking is a stress-reliever, although a life-threatening one. Thus, one of the problems with giving up tobacco is the tense, irritable, edgy feelings you may experience immediately after quitting. To release that tension and nervousness, you may want to try kava for its ability to calm the body and take the edge off. It's certainly worth a try—even though there have been no studies showing that kava helps people quit smoking. At least one quit-smoking program incorporates a kava supplement into its plan—Kick It from LifeScience. In its promotional material, the company says that chiropractors have found an 85 to 95 percent success rate among clients who have tried it. If you consider the devastating effects of smoking on health, kava might be among the best withdrawal aids ever.

EASING ALCOHOL WITHDRAWAL

Today alcohol is the most abused drug in the United States. Ten percent of those who drink alcohol are addicted to it, and ten to twenty percent of all other drinkers are abusers or problem drinkers. Compared to any other commonly used substance, alcohol has one of the lowest "effective dose/lethal dose ratios." In other words there's a very small difference between the amount of alcohol that will get you drunk and the amount that will kill you. But the reason that more people don't die from alcohol intoxication is that the stomach is very sensitive to alcohol and rejects it by vomiting.

Acute alcohol intoxication results in anxiety and irritability, nausea and vomiting, decreased mental functioning, vertigo, coma, and death. Further, chronic alcohol abuse has devastating side effects on every organ in the body, particularly the liver, heart, brain, and muscle and it can thus lead to cancer and diseases of the liver, pancreas, and nervous system. Drinking alcohol in large amounts can also lead to accidents, as well as social, psychological, and emotional problems.

There are many excellent recovery programs for alcoholics. However, for many chronic drinkers who quit suddenly, there is the pain and suffering of the withdrawal process. Withdrawal symptoms include the "shakes" (tremors in the hands), an increase in blood pressure and body temperature, nausea, or diarrhea. These may last from three to five days. Other alcoholics may experience "delirium tremens," or DTs—a serious and often dangerous withdrawal symptom. Extreme tremors, bad dreams, panic attacks, hallucinations, and seizures are among the symptoms of DTs.

Alcohol withdrawal symptoms, including the DTs, are often treated with antianxiety drugs such as benzodiazepines. Such treatment is problematic, however. Some alcoholics get hooked on the drugs and merely trade one addiction for another.

In the early seventies in Vienna, Austria, a research team investigated whether kavain could help alcoholics get through the often-terrifying and painful period of withdrawal. Fifty chronic alcoholics trying to quit drinking were selected for the study, which lasted five weeks. They were divided into two groups: Half were given 200-milligram capsules of kavain, three times a day; the other half received a placebo. Kavain produced good results. Twenty-three of the twenty-five people taking kavain reported that they had far fewer bouts of fear, anxiety, fatigue, dizziness, or nausea. Nearly half the group taking the placebo experienced withdrawal symptoms.

Although this is just one study, it offers a glimmer of hope for people with the disease of alcoholism. Best of all, kava and its components are not addictive—so there's no risk of getting hooked on another substance. If you're an alcoholic seeking to stop drinking, consult your physician before trying kava as a withdrawal aid.

LIFTING YOUR LIBIDO

Has stress invaded your bedroom? If so, kava may be one way to kick it out before your sex life hits a slump—something Oceanian women have known for centuries. In their culture, women would rather their men drink kava than alcohol because when they come home, they want sex.

The truth be told, a loss of interest in lovemaking may be the sign of a deeper problem and certainly requires the help of a qualified counselor. Even so, many couples of all ages are too stressed out to make love on a regular basis—a stress-related celibacy that's a sign of our tension-packed workaday world. Biologically stress produces a temporary drop in the blood levels of sex hormones required for sexual desire, and seriously depletes the libido.

As a proven stress reliever, kava is now being touted as a way to put the magic back in the bedroom. It's not an aphrodisiac by any means, but a way to calm you down and put you in the mood for love. And it does not inter-

fere with coordination or concentration. The only caution: Taking too much kava produces the same effects as
alcohol intoxication, and so would interfere with erotic
interludes.

There is no research supporting kava's use as a sexual
therapeutic aid. However, it has been used by islanders as
an aphrodisiac for thousands of years. Further, some people report that it produces a tingling feeling in the genitalia, heightening the sexual experience.

One manufacturer has already marketed a kava product expressly as a sexual aid. The product is Erotikava,
and it has been featured on *Hard Copy* and *Home and
Family*. Packaged in enticing cobalt blue glass bottles,
the product is a concentrate that you mix with hot water
and drink like tea. Erotikava is formulated with kava
imported from Vanuatu and blended with some Chinese
herbs, which, it is claimed, are also aphrodisiacs.

Kava isn't the first herbal love potion to come along,
however. The search for sexual stimulants is as old as
recorded history. The ancient Greeks, Romans, and Egyptians used garlic as an aphrodisiac. The use of plants as
sexual stimulants is based on an ancient belief that if a
plant looked in any way like human genitalia, then it
possessed sexual vigor. The roots of the mandrake plant,
for example, resemble the human body and in some cases,
the male genitalia. Other herbal aphrodisiacs include
damiana, ginkgo biloba, and yohimbe.

TABLE 2

Traditional Medicinal Uses of Kava in the South Pacific

Country	Medicinal Uses
American Samoa	Urinary infections, gonorrhea
Cook Islands	Urinary infections
Fiji	Laxative, diuretic, diarrhea, lactation aid, asthma, perspiration inducer, contraceptive, sedative
Hawaii	General debility, cold, headache, respiratory diseases, urinary tract infections, joint problems
New Guinea	Sore throat, lactation aid, treatment of cuts, diarrhea
Pohnpei	Gonorrhea
Tahiti	Gonorrhea
Vanuatu	Constipation, conjunctivitis, earache, upset stomach, fever, headaches, weakness, asthma, tuberculosis

Adapted from Lebot, V., M. Merlin, and L. Lindstrom. 1997. *Kava: The Pacific Elixir.* New Haven: Yale University Press.

CHAPTER 11

Kava versus
Prescription Mood Drugs

Emotional distress can strike anyone, at any time. You start feeling anxious, nervous, irritable, sad, depressed, or overwhelmed by daily life. The littlest thing sets you off, you can't sleep, or you want to retreat from the world. In most cases, just talking it out with a friend, a member of the clergy, or someone in your family will ease your mind.

But if your distress hangs around without any sign of ceasing, and you can't do your job or take care of your family—in short, get on with your life—then your troubles could be quite serious and may require professional help, including a combination of psychotherapy and prescription medication.

Medication can effectively reduce the symptoms of anxiety, depression, and other emotional illnesses so that psychotherapy can begin and progress more successfully. Today, as many as 36 million people (roughly 15 percent of all adult Americans) are taking prescription medications daily just for anxiety and its symptoms. The most commonly prescribed drugs are Valium and Xanax. Others include tranquilizers such as BuSpar; tricyclic antidepressants such as Elavil; beta blockers; monoamine oxidase inhibitors such as Nardil, Parnate, and Marplan; and selective serotonin reuptake inhibitors such as Prozac.

Such drugs have worked well for millions of people, restoring their sanity and enabling them to return to productive living. But while the use of drugs to treat anxiety and other emotional disorders can be an effective part of treating and managing the problem, prescription drugs are not without complications. They may alleviate symptoms, but mask underlying problems that ultimately need resolution. Many of these drugs are highly addictive, leading to dependency and abuse. Some increase the risk of accidental injury, interact dangerously with other drugs, and have intolerable side effects.

The risks of drugs in general are beginning to outweigh their benefits. According to a report published in *The Journal of the American Medical Association,* adverse reactions to drugs severe enough to cause death or disability are increasing with alarming frequency. Estimates put the death toll of fatal drug reactions at more than 100,000 deaths annually.

With prescription mood drugs, many people simply do not like the senses-dulling, drugged-out feeling elicited by tranquilizers, sedatives, and antidepressants. Further, more and more people today are uncomfortable taking potentially addictive drugs and prefer nondrug alternatives.

One of those nondrug alternatives is kava. Kava is known to leave your mental sharpness intact, it is not addictive, and it imparts a sense of tranquillity without the worrisome side effects of prescription medications. As an herbal preparation, it works with your body rather than against it (as many prescription drugs do). It's always preferable to try the gentlest, most natural calming agent first.

But how does kava stack up against prescription antianxiety drugs? A couple of landmark studies have looked into this—and the results are quite intriguing. In fact, research supports kava as an effective long-term treatment alternative to benzodiazepines and tricyclic antidepressants.

In a 1990 clinical trial, thirty-eight patients suffering from anxiety were given either oxazepam (Serax), or D,L-kavain (Neuronika), a kava-based drug manufactured in Germany. A benzodiazepine, Serax is commonly used to treat anxiety disorders, as well as anxiety associated with depression. According to *The PDR Family Guide to Prescription Drugs,* its most common side effects include drowsiness; less common or rare side effects include blood disorders, change in sex drive, dizziness, headaches, nausea, skin rashes, and sluggishness. In comparing the patients' responses to the Neuronika versus the Serax, the researchers discovered that both medications reduced anxiety symptoms equally, but that the Neuronika had no adverse side effects.

In a 1993 clinical trial that lasted five days, a kava extract was again compared to Serax. The study involved twelve healthy male volunteers, aged twenty-four to thirty-seven years old. Its goal was to examine what effects, if any, either medication had on memory. While medicated, the volunteers were asked to complete a word recognition exercise. Interestingly, they scored better—that is, remembered more words—when taking the kava extract. Memory performance dipped while taking Serax. Also, kava produced no untoward side effects even though the doses given (200 milligrams three times daily) were quite high.

Kava will not permanently remove stress, anxiety, and depression from your life—nor will prescription drugs. You still have to deal with the root cause. But as these studies show, kava is certainly becoming a viable alternative for dealing temporarily with symptoms before matters become worse.

There may be times, however, when prescription drugs are necessary, and chances are that your physician or psychiatrist will prescribe them. But before you swallow another drug with side effects that could harm you, understand what it does and how it might affect you.

What follows is a discussion of classes of drugs commonly prescribed for emotional disorders, along with their limitations, risks, and precautions.

BENZODIAZEPINES

What Are They? A treatment staple since 1960, benzodiazepines are a class of drugs commonly used to treat general anxiety disorder, phobias, panic attacks, and insomnia. They are among the most widely prescribed drug products in the United States. The most common are diazepam (Valium), chorazepate (Tranxene), oxazepam (Serax), lorazepam (Ativan), and alprazolam (Xanax). Each is more alike than different. They are recommended at specific doses, for short-term use only, and can be effective for helping people get through stress-producing situations. There are approximately thirty-six benzodiazepines sold throughout the world, but only fifteen are approved and marketed for medical use in the United States.

How Do They Work? Benzodiazepines produce their calming effect by interacting with a group of brain cells located in the limbic system, the area of your brain that controls emotions. (Kava acts on the same area of the brain.) First, the drug enters the brain and links up with benzodiazepine "receptors," tiny structures mounted on the surface of cells. Receptors recognize substances and allow their access into the cells. Once inside cells, the benzodiazepines intensify the action of a brain neurotransmitter (a brain chemical that relays messages) called GABA, technically known as gamma-aminobutyric acid. GABA prevents anxiety messages from being transmitted from nerve cell to nerve cell. Valium and Tranxene are fast acting, usually within a half hour, while other benzodiazepines usually act more slowly.

Potential Side Effects: According to *The PDR Family Guide to Prescription Drugs,* the most common side effects include drowsiness, and loss of muscle coordination. Xanax is the least sedating of the benzodiazepines. Each individual benzodiazepine has its own potential side effects, and you should check with your physician and pharmacist for a list.

Long-term and recreational use of benzodiazepines, however, may cause memory impairment, risk of accidents, falls and hip fractures in the elderly, and brain damage, according to scientific research.

Benzodiazepines tend to dull the senses. If taking a benzodiazepine, avoid driving a vehicle, operating machinery, and engaging in any risky activity.

Diazepam (Valium) may block memory formation. In one study, volunteers had trouble recalling word lists and series of numbers they had memorized, either before taking the drug or while under its influence.

According to *The PDR Family Guide to Prescription Drugs,* you can build up a tolerance to benzodiazepines— the need to take higher and higher doses to achieve the same feeling. The risk varies from drug to drug, however. Abrupt withdrawal may cause side effects too. Under the supervision of a physician, you have to withdraw from the drug slowly, in progressively lower doses.

Also worth noting: Studies show that about 21 to 30 percent of patients with generalized anxiety disorder fail to respond to benzodiazepines.

NONBENZODIAZEPINES

What Are They? Some newer drugs labeled nonbenzodiazepines have been developed in recent years. These include zolpidem (Ambien), zopiclone (Imovane), and zaleplon (Sonata). The newest of the trio is zaleplon. Its maker, Wyeth-Ayerst Laboratories, submitted a new drug application to the FDA in February 1998 for the treatment of insomnia in adults and elderly patients.

How Do They Work? Generally, they act on different receptors in the brain than do benzodiazepines and they are designed primarily as sleeping pills.

Potential Side Effects: Studies show that these agents are as effective as benzodiazepines, but with fewer side effects. In its new drug application, Wyeth-Ayerst presented clinical data showing Sonata's effectiveness. In addition, the product was evaluated for safety in more than 2,800 patients with good results.

Check with your physician or pharmacist for information on potential side effects of these medications.

AZAPIRONES

What Are They? This class of drugs is becoming more widely prescribed for treating anxiety. The best known of the group is buspirone (BuSpar), approved in 1986 and effective for patients suffering from generalized anxiety disorder. A plus for buspirone is that it is nonsedating. Tolerance to buspirone does not seem to develop. However, after you discontinue the drug, symptoms may rapidly return. Discontinuing the drug does not cause any withdrawal symptoms. Nor does buspirone have any addictive potential. Other azapirones are in development.

How Do They Work? Buspirone affects the action of the calming neurotransmitter serotonin, which is involved in regulating mood, learning, aggression, sleep, and appetite. Specifically, the drug lowers serotonin levels in people who have too much, and elevates levels in those who have too little (usually people suffering from depression). Studies show that buspirone works as well as the benzodiazepines for managing anxiety, but it has not been found useful for panic attacks. Additionally, buspirone has a low potential for abuse.

Potential Side Effects: According to *The PDR Family Guide to Prescription Drugs,* some of the common side effects may include chest pain, dizziness, dream disturbances, headache, lightheadedness, and nausea.

SELECTIVE SEROTONIN REUPTAKE INHIBITORS (SSRIs)

What Are They? The most famous of these drugs is fluoxetine (Prozac), also among the top-selling drugs of all time. Other SSRIs include paroxetine (Paxil) and sertraline (Zoloft). Other SSRIs are currently in development.

How Do They Work? When you are depressed, there may be a short supply of neurotransmitters (chemical messengers) in your brain. This shortage blocks the transmission of messages between brain cells. Consequently, you feel down, sluggish, apathetic, and often hopeless. SSRIs act only on serotonin, a mood-regulating neurotransmitter. Serotonin levels are linked to feelings of calm and well-being. SSRIs lengthen the amount of time that concentrations of serotonin stay active in the brain, elevating your mood and making you feel better. (The herb St. John's wort appears to do the same.)

SSRIs work as well as other antidepressants, but are better tolerated. Though technically classified as antidepressants, SSRIs are being used with some success to treat anxiety and panic attacks.

Potential Side Effects: According to a 1994 article published in the *Journal of Family Practice,* the most common side effects of SSRIs include nausea, weakness, dizziness, insomnia, sexual difficulties, sweating, tremors, suppressed appetite, and nervousness.

TRICYCLIC ANTIDEPRESSANTS (TCAs)

What Are They? Until Prozac and drugs of its ilk came along, tricyclic antidepressants (TCAs) were the most frequently prescribed medications for depression. Even now, they are preferred by many doctors as the initial medication in the treatment of panic disorder. TCAs have been shown to block panic attacks within three to five weeks, while taking up to ten weeks to alleviate phobic reactions. Drugs in this family include impramine (Tofranil, Janimine), desipramine (Norpramin), and amitriptyline (Elavil, Endep).

How Do They Work? Like most prescription mood drugs, TCAs work on brain chemicals. TCAs, in particular, slow the rate at which certain neurotransmitters—namely serotonin, norepinephrine, and dopamine—reenter the brain. This action increases the concentration of the neurotransmitters throughout the rest of the central nervous system, alleviating feelings of depression.

Potential Side Effects: According to *The PDR Family Guide to Prescription Drugs,* side effects of TCAs include constipation, dizziness, and fatigue. Each type of TCA has its own potential side effects; you should check with your physician or pharmacist for a complete list. If taken in large enough doses, desipramine and amitriptyline can be fatal.

MONOAMINE OXIDASE (MAOs) INHIBITORS

What Are They? MAOs are antidepressants generally reserved for patients with depression accompanied by symptoms of an anxiety disorder. The most commonly prescribed drugs in this group are Nardil, Parnate, and Marplan.

How Do They Work? Monoamine oxidase is an enzyme that destroys serotonin and norepinephrine in the brain. In doing so, this enzyme is neither helpful nor restorative to mental well-being. Thus, by interfering with its action, MAO inhibitors help restore normal mood states. However, these drugs block the enzyme's activity throughout the entire body—an action that can lead to serious, even fatal side effects, especially if these medications are taken with foods containing a substance called tyramine, according to *The PDR Family Guide to Prescription Drugs.* (See below).

MAOs are up to 80 percent effective in treating panic disorder and phobias, but may take up to eight weeks to work. These drugs are usually prescribed for patients who haven't responded to other medications, or who can't use certain other drugs due to medical reasons. For some patients, MAOs are the only antidepressants that make them feel normal again.

Potential Side Effects: Combining MAOs with certain foods or drugs can be dangerous and life threatening. Foods to avoid include beer (even the alcohol-free variety), caffeine, cheese, chocolate, sausage, fava bean pods, liver, pickled foods, spoiled meats or fish, wine, brewer's yeast, and yogurt. MAOs interact dangerously with other drugs, as well. Among them: any kind of diet pill (prescription, nonprescription, and certain types of natural weight-loss supplements); other antidepressants; asthma medications; cold, cough, sinus, and hay fever medications; and nutritional supplements containing l-tryptophan. (Check with your physician or pharmacist for a complete list of foods and drugs to avoid.)

According to *The PDR Family Guide to Prescription Drugs,* side effects include: constipation, dizziness, drowsiness, dry mouth, fatigue, digestive disorders, headache, low blood pressure, and insomnia.

BETA BLOCKERS

What Are They? Beta blockers are actually a family of cardiovascular drugs. The best-known is propanolol (Inderal), which was approved in 1967 to treat irregular heartbeats. Since then, its use has expanded to include the prevention of second heart attacks, plus the treatment of angina, high blood pressure, migraine headaches—and anxiety. The medical profession now looks upon beta blockers as among the most versatile drugs ever discovered.

How Do They Work?   Beta blockers interfere with the action of certain nerve systems in the body that stimulate the activity of the heart, thereby alleviating malfunctions like irregular heartbeats. What's more, they subdue the force and rate of heart contractions. The drugs' action on nerve systems somehow relieves anxiety, although they have no effect on certain symptoms of panic attacks, such as light-headedness, dizziness, and hyperventilation.

Medical experts note that taking a beta blocker one hour before an anticipated stressful event can reduce anxiety significantly. These drugs do not normally produce sedation, nor are they habit-forming.

Potential Side Effects: Beta blockers are not without their side effects. According to *The PDR Family Guide to Prescription Drugs,* these may include: stomach cramps, congestive heart failure, constipation, diarrhea, depression, breathing problems, dry eyes, hair loss, nausea, hallucinations, and several others. See your pharmacist or physician for a full list.

SHOULD YOU TAKE KAVA OR PRESCRIPTION MOOD DRUGS?

Certainly, people who are seriously ill with clinical anxiety or depression will need medication and psychotherapy. Should that medication be herbal or pharmaceutical?

A good rule of thumb is to try the gentler agent first, before resorting to prescription drugs. Do so with the okay of your physician or psychiatrist, however. You can still regulate your own brain chemicals, moods, and stress with natural remedies to handle the ups and downs of life. Kava is one of those agents, and it has many advantages over drugs. For example:

- Kava is not addictive.
- There are no withdrawal problems associated with kava.
- Kava does not interfere with your ability to function at work, nor does it impair memory or mental function.
- Kava does not produce many of the potential side effects you may experience with some prescription mood drugs.

It is important to note, however, that kava does not compare favorably to some drugs in certain respects. For example:

- Kava does not work well if you're suffering from severe depression or anxiety.
- Kava's effects last up to two hours, whereas many prescription mood drugs last much longer.
- Kava does not act as powerfully to relax muscles or prevent convulsions as certain drugs do.

Before you begin drug therapy to treat anxiety, depression, or any other form of emotional distress, discuss the drug, or drugs, with your physician. Ask the following questions:

- Why do I need it?
- How safe is it?
- What are the side effects and how can I minimize them?
- Is the drug addictive or habit-forming?
- Will medication affect my productivity or quality of life?
- How long should I take it?
- What are the long-term consequences of taking this drug?

CHAPTER 12

Kava and Other Calming Herbs

No doubt about it: Stress and anxiety—the tensions and pressures of daily life—wreak havoc with your immune and hormonal systems, lowering your resistance to disease and increasing your chance of being stricken with other illnesses, some of which may be life-threatening (like heart disease and cancer). Stress management and resolution are absolutely vital to your health and to the quality of your life.

Herbs and other natural therapies are now becoming a key pathway to better psychological health. Their relatively safe history of use over thousands of years is comforting when practically every week we read about the dangerous, often fatal side effects of some synthetic drugs.

While kava is now the undisputed champion of herbal calming agents, several other herbs have tranquilizing power, too. Many herbalists recommend that some of these herbs can be used with kava or tried alone, but like kava, all are designed to control your physical response to stress—until you can do something about the stress-causing situation itself.

The herbs in question are black cohosh, California poppy, catnip, chamomile, cramp bark, hops, lemon balm, linden flower, milky oats, motherwort, passionflower, St. John's wort, skullcap, and valerian. They are among the ten thousand herbs used medicinally worldwide.

These herbs can be safely taken with kava and may even work with it synergistically. In herbal medicine, the greatest healing power often comes from a blend of herbs working together in harmony.

One word of warning: Herbs are usually more gentle than prescription drugs, but they still must be used wisely. If you note any unusual reaction to herbal supplementation, seek medical attention quickly.

Here's a rundown on the most frequently used calming herbs, along with their risks and benefits.

BLACK COHOSH

What It Is: Black cohosh (*Cimicifuga racemosa*) grew wild in the Ohio River Valley and was once used by Native American women to treat gynecological problems. In Europe it has been used since the eighteenth century and is today one of the most extensively researched herbs in the treatment of menopause. In menopause, the ovaries no long secrete sufficient amounts of the female hormone estrogen. Hot flashes, backaches, headaches, dizziness, fatigue, irritability, mood swings, nervousness, and insomnia are some of the symptoms of menopause.

Action: Black cohosh contains estrogenic substances that help relieve the symptoms of menopause, particularly hot flashes. But it treats other menopausal symptoms as well, including irritability, mood swings, and sleep disturbances. In one study, menopausal women took forty drops of black cohosh tincture twice a day for six to eight weeks. For irritability, 42.4 percent of the women no longer complained of this problem, and 46 percent no longer experienced mood swings or insomnia. In some studies, black cohosh has proved to be as effective as pharmaceutical estrogen in relieving symptoms. It appears to have a sedative effect, too, and many herbalists now count it among the calming herbs found in nature.

How to Use It:　Black cohosh comes in capsules and tinctures. For best results, follow the manufacturer's suggested usage.

Safety:　Black cohosh has no known harmful side effects and is suitable for long-term use.

CALIFORNIA POPPY

What It Is:　California poppy (*Eschscholzia californica*) is the state flower of California and a popular plant for gardeners. Its brilliant orange cup-shaped flowers make it a stunning plant, one that grows wild on hills, fields, and along roadsides. Except for its roots, the entire plant is used for medicinal purposes.

Action:　California poppy is relatively new on the herbal tranquilizer scene, and there isn't as much research backing it up as there is for herbs like kava and valerian. Nonetheless, scientists do know that it exerts a feeble narcotic effect and depresses the central nervous system. This plant is not to be confused with the poppy that yields opium, since it contains no narcotic derivatives. California poppy looks to be quite promising for easing insomnia and allaying anxiety.

How to Use It: California poppy is available as a tea or in tincture form and can be taken in combination with other calming herbs. To make tea, herbalists recommend using about one teaspoon per cup. If using a tincture, follow the manufacturer's directions for usage. Some herbalists recommend California poppy as an antidote to jet lag. Taking it before your "new" bedtime while traveling, it may help you adjust to a different sleep cycle and help you wake up feeling refreshed.

Safety: As yet, no safety profile has been fully established for California poppy. However, it appears to be relatively safe when taken in recommended amounts for short periods of time.

CATNIP

What It Is: You know it best as the herb that intoxicates your cat, but did you know that it can also have mild tranquilizing effects on humans, too? Catnip, or *Nepeta cataria* as it is known botanically, is a strong-scented herb that is a member of the mint family. The parts of the plant used medicinally are its leaves.

Action: Catnip contains active chemical constituents (nepetalactone isomers) that are similar to the sedative components of valerian and thought to be responsible for the herb's calming qualities. Catnip is a good sleep aid, and it is also sometimes used as a digestive aid and for relief from upset or nervous stomach.

How to Use It: Catnip is usually brewed as a minty but gentle-tasting tea, taken about forty-five minutes prior to retiring. You can drink up to three cups of tea a day. It is also available in supplement form or as an extract. Follow the manufacturer's recommended dosage if you take supplements containing catnip. Herbalists say you should experience stress relief after about one week of taking catnip.

Safety: Catnip is considered by medical authorities to be generally safe when taken in appropriate amounts for short periods of time, but it may interfere with the absorption of iron and other minerals.

CHAMOMILE

What It Is: From a distance, the flowers of chamomile resemble little yellow apples tucked in the grass—which is why the ancient Greeks dubbed the plant *khamaimelon* from *khamai* ("on the ground") and *melon* ("apple"). So prized was chamomile by the ancient Egyptians that they regularly offered it up to their sun god during worship rituals. Also, the Anglo-Saxons considered it one of the nine sacred herbs given to humans by their god Woden. Chamomile is also spelled "camomile."

Chamomile *(Matricaria recutita)* is a member of the daisy family. Ranked as one of the top five herbs used worldwide, it grows in meadows across North America, Europe, North Africa, and parts of Asia. There are several types of chamomile, but the most common is the German variety.

You find chamomile as tea (which is consumed at an estimated rate of a million cups daily), in standardized extracts, and as an ingredient in ointment, lotions, and perfumes.

Action: More than two hundred scientific studies have been conducted on chamomile in the last thirty years, supporting its therapeutic value. Many show that it has a mild sedative effect. Chamomile contains an active compound known as angelic acid, which gives the herb its sedative properties. The herb's chemistry is quite complex, and it works best when taken as a whole herb. As with most herbal remedies, the sum of its chemical components exerts its medicinal action.

Chamomile is also excellent for promoting sleep. In a 1973 study published in the *Journal of Clinical Pharmacology*, twelve patients were given chamomile prior to undergoing a cardiac procedure. Ten of the subjects went into a deep sleep within ten minutes.

In 1997 a research team seeking safer alternatives to benzodiazepines isolated a chemical called apigenin from chamomile and tested it on mice. They discovered that apigenin had a clear antianxiety benefit, based on how it worked in the animals' brains, but did not produce the worrisome sedation you experience with benzodiazepines. The researchers also noted that apigenin is nontoxic and is an anticancer compound. Chamomile as a whole herb has sedative effects, but apigenin by itself does not. Apigenin could thus turn out to be a safe, nonsedating antianxiety agent, if scientists choose to further investigate its potential.

Chamomile has been used to treat a wide range of ailments, including inflammation, muscle spasms, emotionally related gastrointestinal problems, ulcers, toothache, swollen gums, and skin problems. It is known to kill bacteria when applied to the skin.

How to Use It: For use as a sedative or tranquilizer, take up to a gram of the powdered herb as needed. If using an extract, take forty to sixty drops, four times a day as needed. You can consume the tea liberally, without any ill effects. Generally, you may feel the effects of chamomile within an hour.

Safety: Controversy has simmered over whether hay fever sufferers should take chamomile, since it comes from the same botanical family as ragweed. The FDA has told consumers to avoid chamomile if they're allergic to ragweed, while herbalists note that there have been only five documented cases of allergic reactions to the herb. Even so, you may want to approach chamomile cautiously if you are sensitive to ragweed.

CRAMP BARK

What It Is: Like kava, cramp bark (*Viburnum opulus*) is a muscle relaxant, but it has other benefits, too. It acts as a sedative, an anti-inflammatory agent, and a diuretic. Many women take cramp bark to ease menstrual discomforts such as cramps and headaches.

Action: The active ingredient in cramp bark is valeric acid, a sedative. Valeric acid also relaxes the uterine muscle—which is why cramp bark is so effective against menstrual cramps.

How to Use It: Herbalists recommend taking ¼ to 1 teaspoon of cramp bark extract three times a day, with juice or water at mealtime. Or try one capsule of the herb, one to three times a day. You can also brew tea from cramp bark.

Safety: Cramp bark has no known side effects, but should be avoided if you're pregnant or are suffering from any serious disease.

HOPS

What It Is: The ancient Romans grew hops for food, and Europeans began cultivating it more than one thousand years ago to use for brewing beer. Today, hops (*Humulus lupulus*) is used extensively in the brewing industry to give beer its bitter aromatic flavor. Hops has long been prized as a remedy for anxiety and insomnia. It is a member of the mulberry family, and its berries are the part of the plant used medicinally.

Action: Certain chemicals in the plant, lupulin and methylbutenol, are thought to give hops its sedating properties. One study found that a combination product of hops and valerian reduced stress and significantly improved sleep in sleep-disordered patients. Hops is also effective in treating digestive disorders brought on by anxiety.

How to Use It: Herbalists recommend taking hops as a tincture, since this form is more stable. You can also take it as a tea. Follow the manufacturer's recommended dose for usage.

Safety: Hops is considered safe when taken as directed for short periods of time.

LAVENDER

What It Is: Lavender (*Lavandula*) is an herb used to produce lavender oil, commonly used in "aromatherapy." Aromatherapy is the treatment of medical conditions using the scents of highly concentrated oils diffused through the air. Lavender is approved by German Commission E for insomnia.

Action: The aroma of lavender oil has long been known to have a calming effect on the body. In fact animal experiments have found that the herb contains compounds that exert a light sedative effect. Now a recent study has tested this effect on people—with some intriguing results. Researchers from the University of Leicester found that insomniacs in a nursing home slept as well when lavender oil was diffused into the air as they did while taking sleeping pills, including tranquilizers. Further, the people were less restless during sleep than they were while taking drugs. Scientists speculate that sedative compounds in lavender stimulate olfactory nerves in the nose that connect to brain areas that bring on sleep.

Lavender is a fascinating herb. Quite by accident, cancer researchers discovered the anticancer benefits of a family of natural drugs called monterpenes. Among these is perillyl alcohol, found in lavender oil. It appears to regress breast cancer tumors in rats, and preliminary studies in humans are underway in Britain.

How to Use It: You can buy lavender oil and a diffuser at health food stores or at massage therapy clinics. Let several drops of the oil soak into the pad of the diffuser. Insert the pad into the diffuser and plug it into an electrical wall outlet. Within moments, the smell of soothing lavender will fill the room. You can also pour a few drops of the oil into a warm bath or sprinkle it on your bedclothes or sheets. Or, try tucking a lavender sachet inside your pillow at night.

Safety: Aromatherapeutic oils are meant for external use only. Do not ingest lavender oil because it can be toxic if taken internally. The oil is meant to be diffused into the air. When purchasing lavender oil, specify that you want it for sleeplessness. Some lavenders (particularly Spanish lavender) may act as stimulants.

LEMON BALM

What It Is: Grown more than two thousand years ago in Mediterranean areas, this member of the mint family was a food for bees. Even today, beekeepers rub the leaves of this herb over beehives to encourage the insects' productivity. In fact, lemon balm's other name, *Melissa,* is translated from the Latin as "honeybee." Lemon balm's botanical moniker is *Melissa officinalis.*

Action: More by reputation than by scientific knowledge, lemon balm is considered a relaxant to calm anxiety, a sedative to promote sleep, and an antidepressant to combat the blues. Lemon balm contains a biologically active group of chemicals known as terpenes, which are responsible for its sedative action. Lemon balm is approved by the German Commission E as both a sedative and a remedy for nervous stomachs.

Lemon balm is an antiviral as well, considered the first line of herbal defense against herpes sores. This benefit has been validated in scientific studies.

How to Use It: To soothe stress, herbalists recommend drinking up to three cups of lemon balm tea a day. The herb is also available in capsules, which should be taken three times a day or according to the manufacturer's suggested usage, and as an extract (thirty to forty drops daily, four times a day). You may feel relief within a week of regular usage.

Safety: Lemon balm has no known side effects and is considered a relatively safe and gentle herb.

LINDEN FLOWER

What It Is: Linden flower *(Tilia europea)* has long had a reputation as a relaxant and a mood elevator. Its flowers are used for medicinal purposes.

Action: Very little is known about how this herb actually works. A few of its active ingredients have been isolated, and these include oils and sugarlike compounds. Legend has it that one of these sugars possesses the same makeup as the biblical manna.

How to Use It: Linden flower is available as a tea or an extract. Herbalists recommend drinking three cups of the tea daily or supplementing with thirty to forty drops of the extract, four times a day. The herb begins to work within a few days.

Safety: Linden flower has no known side effects and is considered safe when taken in appropriate quantities for short periods of time.

MILKY OATS

What It Is: Milky oats *(Avena sativa)* is the seed of the oat before it has ripened. It is soft and liquidlike—hence the name "milky oats." Herbalists say it is in this stage that the seed yields the highest amount of its active constituents, mainly starches and antioxidant nutrients. The soft seeds are made into tinctures believed to help relieve stress and depression.

Action: There is currently no scientific evidence backing up the mood-elevating value of this herb. Anecdotally, however, people report that it can be used to ease withdrawal from nicotine and that it has a mild stress-relieving effect if taken on a regular basis.

How to Use It: Follow the manufacturer's recommendations for usage.

Safety: Milky oats is a relatively safe herb.

MOTHERWORT

What It Is: Motherwort is an ancient herb believed to settle a mother's womb to aid in delivery—or so seventeenth-century herbalists claimed. Botanically, it is named *cardiaca,* a derivative of the Latin word for heart. In ancient China, the herb was highly prized for its heart-strengthening properties.

Action: Motherwort acts as a mild sedative, eases anxiety, and helps reduce anxiety-related heart palpitations.

How to Use It: Motherwort is sold as a tea, in capsules, and as an extract. For best results, herbalists recommend drinking two cups of the tea daily, take two capsules three times a day, or use thirty to forty drops four times a day. It takes about a week to be effective, and you'll need to use it for at least a month to help relieve anxiety.

Safety: Motherwort should not be taken during pregnancy. Additionally, the herb interferes with normal thyroid function if taken in large doses.

PASSIONFLOWER

What It Is: Passionflower (*passiflora incarnata*) is a perennial vine whose flowers and fruit are made into herbal remedies for treating insomnia, anxiety, and nervousness. In the 1500s, Roman Catholic priests dubbed the plant "passionflower" because they believed that various parts of the plant symbolized aspects of the suffering and death (Passion) of Jesus Christ. Its five petals and five petallike sepals, for example, represented the ten apostles who stayed faithful to Jesus throughout the Passion. Above its petals, the plant features a circle of thin hairs, suggesting the crown of thorns worn by Jesus on the day of His death. Long known to the Aztecs, the plant was discovered in Latin America and is native to the southeastern United States. Passionflower is also called "wild passionflower" and "maypop."

Action: The herb exerts a gentle sedative action and has been found in studies to relieve anxiety, counter insomnia, and reduce high blood pressure. More than forty over-the-counter sedative preparations in the United Kingdom contain passionflower. But the FDA in the United States has banned its use in over-the-counter sedatives because its safety and effectiveness have not been proved according to FDA standards. However, laboratory studies support its use as a sedative, although the exact chemical constituents responsible for its sedative action have not been identified.

A compound called chrysin was recently isolated from

one species of passionflower *(Passiflora coerulea)*. Chrysin is not a sedative but has antianxiety properties. In fact, an experiment found that it was as powerful as Valium, but without the sedating side effects.

How to Use It: Passionflower is available as a dried leaf in capsules, and also as a tincture. It is quite effective when used with other calming herbs, including kava. In fact, it is often a secondary ingredient in many kava products. The German Commission E has officially approved passionflower for nervous anxiety and recommends a dosage of six grams daily. With preparations containing passionflower, follow the manufacturer's directions for dosage.

Safety: Many herbalists believe passionflower is safe when taken as recommended.

SKULLCAP

What It Is: Long ago, herbalists named this perennial herb "skullcap" because its blossoms look like the human skull. A member of the mint family, skullcap goes by other names too: "mad dogweed" (because it was once thought to cure rabies), "blue pimpernel," and "hood wort." Skullcap is known botanically as *Scuttellaria laterifoli*. It grows in Europe, and in the United States from Connecticut to Florida and as far west as Texas.

Action: For more than fifty years, skullcap was considered a sedative by the United States Pharmacopoeia (USP), the organization that sets quality standards for supplements and over-the-counter drugs. Reportedly, skullcap can soothe anxiety, improve sleep, modulate mood swings, and relieve stress-related headaches. Research studies in

China, Europe, and the former Soviet Union have verified its sedating effects. It is rather mild, so you can take it during the day without getting drowsy. Some herbalists recommend it to calm addicts who are withdrawing from narcotics or alcohol. Skullcap's active ingredients include an oil called scutellarin and a glycoside, a type of plant sugar.

How to Take It: This herb is available primarily as a tea. Herbalists recommend drinking one or two cups a day or four cups a day for a stronger dose. Skullcap is also found as a tincture, which you can mix (about thirty to forty drops up to four times a day) in juice or tea. It takes a few weeks of daily use to experience any benefit.

Safety: The herb can be used safely for up to six weeks. However, high doses can cause dizziness or an irregular pulse rate. Skullcap should not be used in conjunction with prescription tranquilizers.

ST. JOHN'S WORT

What It Is: On the herbal center stage for several years now is St. John's wort, a common herb grown throughout Europe and North America. Translated, the word *wort* is Old English for "plant." Its botanical name, *hypericum,* comes from a Greek word meaning "over an apparition." The herb was believed to be so obnoxious that it would cause evil spirits to fly away. In the Middle Ages, peasants burned the herb on St. John's Day (June 24) to rid the air of demons.

Although it has been around for ages—the Greeks and Romans used it to treat infections and inflammation—St. John's wort has been a much publicized topic in the media. In 1997 German and American researchers evaluated twenty-three studies of St. John's wort and concluded that it worked as well as, and sometimes better than, prescription antidepressants for treating mild to moderate depression, a mental disorder that affects one out of every four Americans. Best of all, the herbal treatment produced fewer side effects.

Action: St. John's wort is believed to increase serotonin levels in the brain, although no one knows exactly how. Elevated serotonin levels tend to improve mood.

The active compound in St. John's wort is hypericin, a chemical that was first isolated from the herb in 1942 and provides a significant antidepressant effect. Supplementing with St. John's wort relieves depression, elevates mood, calms anxiety, provides an increased sense of well-being, and enhances sleep.

Some pharmacologists think other active ingredients besides hypericin may be at work, too. One of these is called hyperforin. In a double-blind, placebo-controlled study, patients with mild to moderate episodes of depression responded positively to a St. John's wort extract that had been fortified with extra hyperforin. Seventy-two people participated in the study. Half the group took 300 milligrams of the supplement three times a day; the other half took a placebo. In just two weeks, those taking the fortified extract experienced significant drops in their depressive feelings. Nature's Way markets a hyperforin-rich St. John's wort in the United States under the Perika label. The product is standardized to contain 3 percent hyperforin.

How to Use It: The usual dosage is two capsules daily (200 to 300 milligrams) of a capsulated product standardized to 3 percent hypericin. It takes about two to four weeks for the herb to take effect. Unlike many prescription antidepressants, there are no withdrawal symptoms from discontinuing the use of St. John's wort. Nor is the herb addictive.

Safety: A side effect that has been noted with St. John's wort is weight gain. The herb can also make your skin more sensitive to light. This means you'll be more likely to get a sunburn if outside. If you're fair skinned and supplementing with St. John's wort, avoid sunlight.

St. John's wort has been used extensively in Germany with no published reports of serious side effects. Observations on 3,250 patients taking the supplement noted that the most common side effects were gastrointestinal symptoms (0.6 percent), allergic reactions (0.5 percent), and fatigue (0.4 percent).

The herb should not be taken in conjunction with other drugs that affect serotonin levels, such as fluoxetine (Prozac) and monoamine oxidase (MAO) inhibitors. If taken with these drugs, serious side effects could result, including high blood pressure and a dangerous condition called the serotonin syndrome. This syndrome is marked by sweating, agitation, upset stomach, and jerky muscles. Severe reactions cause seizures, coma, and even death.

As with any supplement, do not take St. John's wort if you are pregnant, nursing, or suffering from any disease. Antidepressants such as St. John's wort should be taken under medical supervision.

VALERIAN

What It Is: Until kava came along, valerian was the herb of choice for jangled nerves. Used by Hippocrates as early as the fourth century, valerian *(Valeriana officinalis)* is a perennial herb that often grows to more than five feet high, with an attractive spray of pink or white flowers. In some areas of New England, valerian is a roadside weed. The parts of the plant used for medicinal purposes are the roots and rhizome. The herb has a very offensive odor and in fifth century Greece, ancient physicians dubbed it *Phu,* which not coincidentally is a root of our word, "pew." Its current name, "valerian," comes from the Latin word, *valere,* meaning "to be in health." Even though its name sounds like "Valium," there's no relation. Valerian goes by other names, too: "setwell," "herba benedicta," and "amantila."

Beginning in the 1700s, most European dispensaries listed valerian as a treatment for nervous ailments, including hysteria and insomnia. Today in Germany alone, more than 150 drugs are made from valerian root. Until 1942 valerian was listed as an official drug by the United States Pharmacopoeia. Today it is approved as a food (as most herbs are) but not as a drug. Available without a prescription, valerian comes in capsules, tablets, teas, and tinctures and is often formulated with other calming herbs, such as kava, hops, passionflower, or skullcap.

Action: For more than thirty years, more than two hundred scientific studies on valerian's constituents have been published in medical literature, particularly in Europe. As noted above, one study found that a combination product of hops and valerian was an effective stress reducer and sleep inducer. Overall, valerian has a gentle, mild tranquilizing effect.

In fact, valerian is the most widely studied herb for the treatment of insomnia. In medical experiments, valerian has been found to work as well as benzodiazepines or barbiturates to treat insomnia. Many people report "perfect sleep" after supplementing with valerian. Additionally, the herb reduces "sleep latency," the time it takes to fall asleep after your head hits the pillow.

Approximately 120 chemicals have been identified in valerian. Numerous animal studies have shown that extracts of these chemicals depress the central nervous system and thus may be antidepressants. Even so, scientists are not sure which chemicals are biologically active and responsible for this effect. As with most herbs, however, it is the synergistic action of many chemical components that most likely produces valerian's sedative effect.

Valerian is notable, too, in that alternative medicine experts believe it may help people break their addiction to prescription tranquilizers. In Europe it is used to treat addictions to some benzodiazepines.

Additionally, valerian confers benefits on the heart. It contains antiarrhythmic compounds, helps lower blood pressure, increases blood flow to the heart, and enhances the heart's ability to pump blood. (As with any herb or natural supplement, check with your physician before taking valerian for any medical condition.)

How to Use It: Herbalists suggest the following usage: capsules or tablets, up to six a day; extract, twenty to thirty drops four times a day. (As a general rule of thumb, it's advisable to follow the manufacturer's recommended dose.) Valerian is available as a tea, too, but it has an earthy, pungent, and rather unpleasant taste. If you can stand it, try drinking a cup of valerian tea about a half hour before going to bed to treat insomnia.

Hops and lemon balm work well with valerian, too, especially as remedies for sleeplessness.

Like kava, valerian has virtually no aftereffects. It usually leaves you feeling refreshed rather than sluggish. If you feel you're not responding to valerian, herbalists recommend slightly increasing the amount you're using, but you'll get a slight headache if you take too much.

Safety: Medical authorities consider valerian relatively safe when taken in recommended quantities for no more than two or three weeks. The herb is certainly a superior first-choice course of action before resorting to prescription sedatives and tranquilizers.

A problem with valerian is that its active chemicals can vary in potency and concentration from plant to plant. Thus, valerian products may also vary in strength. You may have to experiment with various doses to get the desired effect.

Very high doses (over recommended amounts), however, can cause headaches, excitability, heart disturbances, muscular spasms, and, paradoxically, insomnia. There is some preliminary evidence that long-term overusage of valerian may cause liver damage.

COMBINATION FORMULAS

Many companies are marketing multiherb formulations for the treatment of insomnia, stress, and anxiety. A few studies have been done on such formulations, mostly in Europe where herbal medicine is widely practiced and accepted. In 1997 a group of French researchers published a study on a product named Euphytose, which contains the mild sedatives hawthorn, black horehound, passionflower, and valerian, and the stimulant herbs kola nut and guarana. Coordinated by psychiatrists, the study investigated how well Euphytose alleviated anxiety in a group of 182 patients. For a period of twenty-eight days, half the patients took Euphytose; the other half, a placebo. By the end of the study, anxiety symptoms in patients on Euphytose had dropped dramatically, compared to those taking the placebo.

A German study published in 1996 compared the morning-after (hangover) effects of two plant-based sleep remedies (a valerian/hops formula and a valerian syrup) with flunitrazepam (a tranquilizer). The researchers found that the tranquilizer significantly impaired mental alertness the next morning and constituted a potential hazard, while the plant remedies affected alertness only slightly. However, those who took the herbal preparations said they felt more alert and active the next day. Flunitrazepam (Rohypnol), incidentally, is the most abused benzodiazepine drug in Europe, Asia, and Oceania, causing paranoia, amnesia, dependence, and death, according to the FDA. It is not marketed in the United States at this time.

An earlier study conducted in Germany by the same lead researcher compared the potential side effects of bromazepam (a tranquilizer that is not currently marketed in the United States) to those of Valverde, an herbal preparation containing valerian, lemon balm, passionflower, and pestilence wort. The researchers expected bromazepam to have more side effects, such as sedation and impairment of alertness, than the herbal supplement would have. But neither produced any side effects at all.

GENERAL GUIDELINES FOR USING HERBAL SEDATIVES AND TRANQUILIZERS

1. Herbal treatments for anxiety, stress, depression, and other mood disorders should be considered temporary treatments. Avoid habitual use.

2. Long-term improvement of mood disorders should come from professional therapy and spiritual growth, not from dependence on herbal remedies or prescription drugs.

3. Do not take any herbs if you are pregnant or lactating.

4. Educate yourself on herbal therapies and the research, if any, behind them.

5. Purchase herbal supplements from well-known, reputable companies.

6. Read the labels on any herb you might purchase. Make sure you know what each ingredient is and what effect it has on the body. Don't buy the supplement until you have learned all you can about its ingredients and its potential side effects.

7. Tell your doctor you are taking an herbal supplement, especially during an illness or before surgery, or if you have a preexisting medical condition. If you don't communicate this information, there is a risk that your doctor will unwittingly prescribe something that will interact dangerously with the supplement.

8. Follow the manufacturer's or doctor's suggestion regarding dosage. Also, pay close attention to any warnings or precautions that appear on the supplement label.

9. Report any adverse effects to your physician.

10. As with medicines, regard any herb as potentially harmful to children and keep them safely out of sight.

CHAPTER 13

Other Natural
Tension-Tamers

If you'd love to soothe jangled nerves, or chase the blues, there is another category of natural supplements worth a try: vitamins, minerals, and amino acids. Several of these nutrients do wonders for anxiety disorders and depression. Plus they can be taken if you're already using kava and other calming herbs, since there's no apparent interaction. Here's a closer look.

B-COMPLEX VITAMINS

This is a family of nutrients that includes eight major vitamins—thiamine, riboflavin, niacin, vitamin B_{12}, pyridoxine, folic acid, pantothenic acid, and biotin, along with some "minor" B vitamins such as inositol and choline. These work in accord to ensure proper digestion, metabolism, and energy production. Several are of extreme importance to mental health.

INOSITOL

Though not considered a full-fledged member of the B-complex family, inositol has numerous duties in the body. It is involved in fat metabolism and is required for cell growth in the bone marrow, eye membranes, and intestines.

Inositol is critical to brain-cell chemistry and used by various types of receptors to help transmit messages. With the exception of niacin, there is more inositol in the body than any other vitamin. However, levels of inositol are lower than normal in the cerebrospinal fluid of depressed patients. This discovery prompted researchers to study inositol's benefit in treating depression. In a 1995 study patients who took twelve grams daily of inositol for four weeks experienced a significantly greater reduction in depressive symptoms than patients who took a placebo.

So compelling was this finding that some of the same researchers decided to investigate inositol's value in treating panic disorder. They recruited twenty-one patients with panic disorder, with or without agoraphobia, and treated them with twelve grams a day of inositol or a placebo for four weeks. Again, the results were promising. The inositol-treated group had fewer panic attacks, and when they did have a panic attack, it was less severe. Plus, the severity of their agoraphobia declined significantly. Little change was observed in the placebo group. The researchers concluded that "the fact that inositol is a natural component of the human diet makes it a potentially attractive therapeutic for panic disorder."

There's more. Their research continued with a look into whether inositol could help people suffering from obsessive-compulsive disorder. In 1996 thirteen patients with this disorder were given eighteen grams of inositol daily, or a placebo, for six weeks. Remarkably, inositol significantly helped obsessive-compulsive sufferers, too.

Why does inositol work so well in treating depression, panic disorder, and obsessive-compulsive disorder? Inositol appears to act on the same areas of the brain as do Prozac and other selective serotonin reuptake inhibitors, somehow regulating normal levels of the brain chemical serotonin. And the other incredible news about inositol is that it produces no untoward side effects.

Inositol is certainly worth looking at if you're plagued by any of these disorders. It is available as a supplement and also found in whole grains, citrus fruits, brewer's yeast, and liver. You get about a gram of inositol a day from food.

FOLIC ACID

Folic acid is the vitamin that with the help of vitamin B_{12} helps produce red blood cells in the bone marrow. Found in green leafy vegetables, legumes, and whole grains, it also helps reproducing cells synthesize proteins and genetic material.

Folic acid first attracted attention for its role in pregnancy. During pregnancy, folic acid helps create red blood cells for the increased blood volume required by the mother, fetus, and placenta. So important is folic acid intake to women in their childbearing years that foods are now being fortified with it.

There is renewed excitement over folic acid because of its protective role against heart disease and cancer. The vitamin reduces homocysteine, a proteinlike substance, in the tissues and blood. High homocysteine levels have been linked to heart disease. And recent scientific experiments have revealed that folic acid may prevent the formation of precancerous lesions that could lead to cervical cancer.

A short supply of folic acid is commonly found in people suffering from depression and other psychiatric disorders such as dementia and schizophrenia. Abnormally low stores of folic acid reduce levels of brain chemicals involved in regulating your moods. Also, sufficient folic acid is needed to fight homocysteine, which can be poisonous to brain cells, causing them to self-destruct.

Scientists who have studied the relationship between folic acid and mental functioning recommend that the vitamin be given to patients suffering from unipolar or bipolar depression, as well as to geriatric patients with dementia, as a complement to their regular therapy. As little as 400 micrograms daily have been found to relieve depression in people with a diagnosed folic acid deficiency. That's the level found in most multiple vitamins.

Stress, disease, and alcohol consumption all increase your need for folic acid. Make sure you're getting 400 to 800 micrograms a day of this vitamin.

VITAMIN B$_5$ (PANTOTHENIC ACID)

The name pantothenic acid comes from the Greek word *pantothen,* which means "everywhere"—a fitting translation because this B-complex vitamin is present in every living cell. First recognized as a substance that stimulates growth, pantothenic acid has been called an "anti-stress vitamin." This is because pantothenic acid stimulates the adrenal glands and boosts production of important stress-coping hormones. Chronic stress can cause a shortage of pantothenic acid, exhausting the adrenal glands and hindering their ability to produce these hormones.

Foods rich in pantothenic acid include organ meats, brewer's yeast, egg yolks, and whole grains. Cooking and food processing destroy up to 50 percent (sometimes more) of the vitamin.

Pantothenic acid is so widespread in foods, however, that deficiencies are usually not a problem. In addition, the vitamin can be made in the body by intestinal bacteria. Many multivitamin supplements also contain pantothenic acid. The recommended daily intake for adults is four to seven milligrams daily.

VITAMIN B$_{12}$

Vital to healthy blood and a normal nervous system, vitamin B$_{12}$ is the only vitamin found primarily in animal products. It works in partnership with folic acid to form red blood cells in the bone marrow.

Deficiencies can produce memory problems, depression, psychosis, and schizophrenia. The older you get, the greater your risk of suffering from a vitamin B$_{12}$ deficiency. That's because your ability to absorb the nutrient declines with age due to "atrophic gastritis," the inability to secrete enough stomach acid to kill off bacteria.

As many as 25 to 30 percent of people age sixty-five and 40 percent of eighty-year-olds suffer from this problem. Bacteria lingers in the stomach and upper part of the small bowel, blocking the absorption of vitamin B$_{12}$ and other nutrients. This can lead to worrisome deficiencies. An insufficiency of vitamin B$_{12}$ can cause a buildup of homocysteine. High homocysteine levels have been linked to mental impairment and heart disease.

Fortunately, vitamin B$_{12}$ supplements are easily absorbed by the body—even if you have atrophic gastritis. Research indicates that taking 500 to 1,000 micrograms daily is sufficient for older people to curb malabsorption problems. Vitamin B$_{12}$ isn't toxic either, even in high doses.

Some vegetarians may be at risk of a vitamin B_{12} deficiency, too. If you're a vegetarian who does not eat animal foods, be sure to get enough vitamin B_{12}. Fermented and cultured foods such as tempeh and miso contain some B_{12}; so do vegetarian foods fortified with the nutrient. The best approach is to supplement with a multiple vitamin containing the RDA of vitamin B_{12} (six micrograms).

VITAMIN C

Vitamin C maintains collagen, helps create red blood cells, promotes wound healing, fights bacterial infection, and protects eyes against the oxidative damage that leads to cataracts.

Vitamin C has also been dubbed the "anti-stress vitamin." When hormones flood your system in response to prolonged stress or anxiety, vitamin C is depleted. Thus, you need more vitamin C when you're under stress.

Current research shows that taking 250 milligrams a day provides enough protection. But if you take 500 milligrams a day, vitamin C may block your body's use of other nutrients. Levels higher than 1,000 milligrams a day can harm your immune system by interfering with the activity of disease-fighting white blood cells.

Vitamin C is found in tomatoes, citrus fruits, strawberries, green peppers, potatoes, and dark green vegetables.

MAGNESIUM

Nutritionists have long known that the typical American diet is low in magnesium, a mineral that is involved in many energy-producing reactions. Magnesium is required to manufacture certain relaxant hormones, which are involved in reducing the anxiety and mood swings common in premenstrual syndrome.

Here is something else to consider: People who exhibit type A behavior (usually aggressive and sometimes hostile) are at risk of a magnesium deficiency. Their bodies produce higher levels of stress hormones that ultimately cause cells to lose magnesium. This deficiency has implications for heart health. Heart cells, in particular, need a sufficient supply of magnesium. The magnesium-robbing effect of stress could damage the heart muscle—which is one possible explanation for the high rate of cardiovascular problems among type A people.

Magnesium-rich foods include chickpeas, beet greens, and turnip greens. The recommended daily allowance (RDA) for magnesium is 350 milligrams for adult men and 280 milligrams for adult women.

PHENYLALANINE

The amino acid, phenylalanine, is a building block for certain brain neurotransmitters. It has sometimes been used to treat depression because it provides an amphetaminelike boost in mood. In one study, twenty patients received between 75 and 200 milligrams of phenylalanine daily for twenty days. At the end of the study period, twelve patients were mentally well enough to be discharged from the hospital. Other research indicates that phenylalanine may be effective in treating bipolar depression, and some physicians feel that it can be used safely in conjunction with some mood drugs. In at least one study, phenylalanine was found comparable to imipramine (Tofranil) in reducing symptoms of depression. Imipramine is a tricyclic antidepressant used to treat depression.

This amino acid is also believed to favorably affect

memory and alertness. And because of its ability to preserve endorphins (the body's natural painkillers), phenylalanine has also been used for pain relief.

Phenylalanine is found naturally in almonds, avocados, bananas, cheese, cottage cheese, nonfat dried milk, chocolate, pumpkin seeds, and sesame seeds.

The form in which this supplement is usually found is dl-phenylalanine. Follow the manufacturer's recommendations for dosage. Vitamin C and vitamin B_6 are required for the conversion of phenylalanine into neurotransmitters. Thus, supplementing with both vitamins is often recommended when taking phenylalanine.

Phenylalanine should be avoided by anyone taking antidepressants; anyone suffering from high blood pressure, the genetic illness phenylketonuria (PKU), diabetes, or migraine headaches; and anyone being treated for melanoma, a serious form of skin cancer. The supplement could aggravate these conditions. You shouldn't supplement with isolated amino acids for longer than a few weeks. Amino acid supplementation is not a substitute for medical evaluation and treatment for depression.

TYROSINE

Tyrosine is an amino acid made from phenylalanine and it is a building block of norepinephrine and dopamine, two good-mood brain chemicals. Chronic stress depletes these important chemicals. But in a dramatic nutritional rescue, supplementing with tyrosine appears to prevent this depletion, thus making the amino acid a good antidote to stress.

Like its counterpart phenylalanine, tyrosine has been used to relieve depression and increase mental alertness. In fact, the United States military has investigated using tyrosine to reduce the symptoms of stress among soldiers—symptoms such as anxiety, poor moods, fatigue, and performance problems. In one study, investigators found that tyrosine (100 milligrams daily per kilogram of body weight) reversed the physiological and psychological symptoms of stress. Tyrosine, like phenylalanine, has been compared to imipramine in tests, but found not to work as well.

Tyrosine may help treat narcolepsy, a sleep disorder in which sufferers involuntarily fall asleep during the day. The disorder is thought to be linked to abnormal levels of the brain chemical, dopamine. When eight narcoleptics were treated daily with 100 milligrams of tyrosine per kilogram of body weight, they were free from daytime sleep attacks after six months of treatment. The researchers noted that "tyrosine offers a valuable new approach to the management of narcolepsy." However, another study produced the opposite results. More research is needed to confirm whether tyrosine is beneficial for this particular sleep disorder.

Tyrosine is found naturally in almonds, avocados, bananas, cheese, lima beans, and pumpkin seeds.

Follow the manufacturer's recommendation for dosage. Vitamins C and B_6 are involved in converting tyrosine into neurotransmitters, so supplementing with these vitamins is often recommended.

Do not supplement with tyrosine if you're taking beta-blocker drugs or antidepressants or suffering from high blood pressure (tyrosine may cause blood pressure to rise even higher). If you're allergic to any foods containing tyrosine, do not supplement. Additionally, you shouldn't supplement with isolated amino acids such as tyrosine or phenylalanine for longer than a few weeks.

KAVA AND NUTRITIONAL SUPPLEMENTS

If you're pursuing a natural course for treating your mood disorder, you might consider taking kava in addition to supplements. However, be aware that such combination therapy has not been formally researched. Be sure to get the approval of your physician before embarking on a supplement program to fight stress and improve your mood.

CHAPTER 14

What You Should Know about Taking Kava:

How Much, What Kind, Where to Buy

If you're ready to relax, or relieve stress, tension, and other emotional problems naturally, here are guidelines and purchasing pointers for supplementing with kava.

KAVA: FIGURING OUT HOW MUCH TO TAKE

Kava varies in its potency—for several reasons:

Varieties of Kava. Scientists have analyzed kava roots taken from different regions of the South Pacific to compare the concentrations of their active constituents. Kava from Vanuatu, for example, is much stronger than kava from Fiji. Samoan kava is considerably less potent than kava cultivated in other parts of Oceania.

Maturity. The age of the root makes a difference in its strength. The older the root, the more potent its kavalactones. Reportedly, too, some herbal manufacturers produce their kava products from the leaves of the plant, which contain fewer kavalactones than the root does.

Modern Preparation Methods. Preparing a cold infusion by steeping the dried root in cold water produces a much stronger dose than taking kava in capsule or extract form.

Shelf Life. Kava products don't retain their potency forever. There is one study that has been conducted on the stability of kavalactones, and it found that dry powdered root, stored at room temperature, will degrade over a three-year period. Hence, any powdered product, including capsules, will gradually lose potency over time.

KAVA DOSAGES

Kava capsules come in different potencies, ranging from 100 to 250 milligrams per capsule. Kavalactones (the active ingredients in kava) in the capsules can vary in concentration from 30 to 70 percent. If you take a 100-milligram capsule containing a 30-percent kava extract, for example, you'll ingest 30 milligrams of kavalactones ($.30 \times 100$).

Compared to kava pills, ready-to-use kava powder is much more concentrated in kavalactones and thus quite strong. On average, three grams of dried root powder contain 300 milligrams of kavalactones. However, the labels of many powder products do not indicate the percent of kavalactones contained in each dose. This makes it hard to know how much you're taking in.

Given the variation in effect and strength of various kava products, how much should you take? If you've never used kava before, consider following the German Commission E recommendation of 60 to 120 milligrams of kavalactones daily. Or abide by the supplement manufacturer's recommended dosage as listed on the product label.

You might want to tailor your dosage to treat a specific condition, however. To help you, here are some general dosage guidelines that are frequently recommended by health care professionals who specialize in herbal medicine:

General stress: up to 240 milligrams of kavalactones daily.

Anxiety: up to 300 milligrams of kavalactones daily.

Depression: 180 milligrams of kavalactones daily.

Insomnia: 200 milligrams of kavalactones, taken thirty to sixty minutes before going to bed.

Alcohol withdrawal: 200 milligrams of kavain extract three times a day. (Alcohol withdrawal should be done under the care and supervision of a physician.)

Be sure to discuss dosages with your physician or health care professional.

KAVA PRECAUTIONS

Observe how you feel after taking kava, watching for any unusual reactions. If you have an adverse reaction, discontinue the supplement. Fortunately, though, side effects from moderate, short-term kava use are virtually nonexistent.

Unless under medical supervision, do not supplement with kava for longer than three months at a time. Neither should you take kava while on prescription mood medications as this may lead to possibly dangerous interactions. One study found that a patient lapsed into a near comatose state due to an interaction with kava and alprazolam (Xanax). Do not take kava with any benzodiazepine tranquilizers such as those discussed in chapter 11. To avoid possibly dangerous interactions, you should not take kava with alcohol or antihistamines such as Benadryl.

And, of course, it's not a good idea to operate a vehicle or to do any activities requiring a fast reaction time while you're taking kava.

The bottom line is that you must treat kava as medication. In other words, respect it.

COMING TO TERMS WITH SUPPLEMENTS

If you're ready to go kava shopping, it's a good idea to master some herbal language first. It will help you buy the right formulation for your needs and possibly get a better deal on your purchase. Also, understanding the lingo will help you become a better label reader. Here goes:

CAPSULES

Capsules contain the dried root powder, often in a base of complementary herbs. The popular kava product, Kavatrol, for example, comes in a base of other calming herbs, including passionflower, chamomile, and hops. An advantage of the capsule form is its convenience. You don't have to mix the kava in water or strain it through mesh. Capsules, of course, do not have the unpleasant earthy taste of liquid preparations, but may take longer to assimilate in the body.

EXTRACTS

An extract is an herb that has been broken down or processed so that more of its active ingredients are used in the product. The extraction process may involve dissolving the herb in water, alcohol, or a solvent to obtain the active ingredients. An extract may or may not be "standardized." (See page 175.)

COLD EXTRACT

This is a method in which an herb is prepared with cold water, which helps preserve the biologically active ingredients. With some kava products, it is necessary to first mix the dry kava powder in cold water, strain the mixture through a fine mesh cloth, then squeeze the cloth to extract as much of the "juice" or kava-concentrated liquid as possible. This method is similar to the way fresh kava is prepared traditionally on South Pacific islands.

INFUSION

An infusion is a way of preparing herbs that is similar to making tea. Infusions are generally used to prepare the leaves and flowers of an herb. You boil water first, remove it from the heat, then add the herb. Let the mixture sit for ten to twenty minutes (or until it has cooled off) to extract the active ingredients. Next, strain off the plant material and drink the beverage cool or lukewarm, or gently reheat it. A downside of fixing kava in this manner is that the active ingredients in the herb are vulnerable to heat and may lose some of their potency.

DECOCTION

A decoction is similar to an infusion, only you boil the plant material directly in the water (usually for about ten to twenty minutes). Boiling in this manner effectively forces the plant material to give up its active components and works best with hard materials such as roots and barks. So if you buy dry kava root chunks, you might want to try this method.

TEA

Like an infusion, tea is prepared by steeping the dried root material in hot water. Kava extracts can be made into tea also. Simply place a few dropperfuls of the extract into hot water. But keep in mind that heat may sap some of the kava's strength.

TINCTURE

Tinctures are made in a number of ways, but the most common is to steep the dry herb in a mixture of water and a solvent (usually alcohol). Alcohol extracts the biologically active constituents from the herb, stabilizes and preserves them. After a few days, the mixture is strained, leaving a concentrated form of the herb. Many companies produce glycerin-based tinctures, which are alcohol free. These are preferable if you wish to avoid alcohol.

STANDARDIZED

This term means the products have been processed to ensure a uniform level of one or more isolated active ingredients from batch to batch. To standardize a product, the manufacturer extracts key active ingredients from the whole herb, measures them, sometimes concentrates them, and then formulates them in a base with other nutrients, including the whole herb.

Standardization is a good guarantee that the product contains the exact amounts to produce the desired results. To check that a product carries this assurance, you must read the labels and look for the ingredients that have been standardized.

MICRONIZED

"Micronized" describes herbs that have been pulverized into ultrafine particles. A company named Better Living Products, Inc. (www.betterlivingusa.com) developed the process for "micronizing" kava root—a process that apparently releases kavalactones normally discarded by other processing methods. The result is an ultrafine powder you can easily mix with water or in any kind of smoothie-type drink. With micronized kava root, there's no need to filter out any plant particles using mesh cloth.

PHARMACEUTICAL GRADE

This is a term you may encounter on some kava products. It means the kava has been purchased from a reputable pharmaceutical company. The label "pharmaceutical grade" is supposed to signify that the product is pure.

READY-TO-DRINK

This term describes supplements available as beverages or soft drinks. Just pop the lid or top and swill it down. Among their advantages: convenience, taste, and rapid absorption by the body.

Ready-to-drink beverages, teas, and soft drinks formulated with kava have become wildly popular. A company named Daily Wellness markets a kava drink called Stress Soother, launched in 1997 as part of its Elix line of ready-to-drink herbal and vitamin supplements available at health and natural food stores nationwide.

Made with a base of herbal black and green teas, a citrus-flavored carbonated beverage called XTZ Tea contains kava, along with two caffeine-containing herbs, guarana and kola. You can order this product from Only Gourmet at its web site, www.onlygourmet.com. Or you can call 1–888–41–FOODS to order by telephone. The distributor accepts Visa, MasterCard, American Express, Visa Cash, and check.

Relaxation Cocktail is one of five beverages in a line of ready-to-drinks called Tribal Tonics, from Apple & Eve L.P. It's a natural herbal supplement made with green tea, cane juice, and standardized herbal extracts. Specifically, it contains 75 milligrams of kava (standardized to 40 percent kavalactones), 100 milligrams chamomile (another calming herb), beta carotene, hawthorn berry, and citric acid. The manufacturer plans to donate 5 percent of its profits to the promotion and protection of various native groups, including the people of Vanuatu, the tiny South Pacific republic that supplies the kava for Relaxation Cocktail. In Vanuatu, proceeds will be used to help cover the costs of a national vaccination program. Available in 11.5-ounce recyclable cans, 16-ounce glass bottles, and four-packs, Tribal Tonics are sold in convenience, grocery, specialty, and natural food outlets in the United States.

Hansen Functionals makes a line of herbal beverages, including D-Stress, a carbonated drink formulated with kava (100 milligrams). Other herbs in the drink include St. John's wort (100 milligrams) and chamomile (100 milligrams). D-Stress boasts that it "contributes to a relaxed feeling of general well-being during times of physical and mental stress." A warning label alerts drinkers to "exercise caution when driving a motor vehicle or operating machinery." You can usually find the product in health food stores.

Kava Kaze and Kava Sutra, manufactured by Weird Pop of Britain, are among the rapidly growing brands of kava drinks. Kava Kaze contains a combination of several herbs besides kava: ginseng, ginkgo, ginger, guarana, green tea, and nutmeg. Kava Sutra is similar in formulation, but has a fruity taste. No food coloring or preservatives are used in either drink. People who have tried these beverages rave about them. As one person commented about Kava Sutra: "It's really subtle but you can sense that it really works." Both products are distributed by Real Soda in Real Bottles, Ltd. For information on where to buy them, you can call the distributor at 310–326–9202, or 310–326–7951 (fax), or access the distributor's web site at www.realsoda.com.

If you want to learn more about herbal-based beverages and soft drinks, access BevNet at www.bevnet.com/reviews, where you'll find critiques of nonalcoholic beverages. Founded in 1996, BevNet is an organization that tests soft drinks and provides written reviews of them on the World Wide Web. Herbal sodas, including those containing kava, are reviewed regularly.

SPRAY

Sprays are a rather new type of "delivery system" for supplements and are reportedly better absorbed than injections, sublingual (under the tongue) methods, transdermal patches, and pills taken orally. A few kava spray products are now available on the market. You simply squirt the mist under your tongue—and the kava goes right into your system. Convenient to carry in your purse or pocket, kava sprays are usually flavored with mint or other flavorings to mask kava's usually muddy taste.

BATH THERAPY

Yes, can you believe it? Kava comes in a bath product! Natural Sports Bath, made by Aubrey Organics, is an herbal bath emulsion to which kava and other herbs have been added. If you have achy muscles after a hard workout or strenuous physical labor, you might want to try such a product.

Kava's pain-relieving, muscle-relaxing properties are thought to go to work right in the bathtub, penetrating the skin to soothe minor body aches and tired, sore muscles. Herbal baths are a form of "hydrotherapy"—the use of water to treat illness. Hydrotherapy is nothing new—

even Hippocrates recommended it. It has long been popular in Europe where it is quite common to add minerals or herbs to the water for a healing effect.

OTHER KAVA PRODUCTS

In addition to these products, supplement and food manufacturers see more uses for kava. There are already kava corn chips in some markets, and you can buy a product called Happy and Healthy Chocolate Chip Cookies baked with kava, St. John's wort, ginkgo biloba, and a weight-control herb called garcinia cambogia. Products such as kava chewing gum, kava toothpaste, and kava coffee may not be too far off.

EUROPEAN KAVA PRODUCTS

In Europe, at least seventeen different kava preparations are available on the market. One of these is Laitan, the only pure kava product, billed as "The New Phytotherapeutic Remedy for nervous anxiety, tension, and restlessness." It comes in capsules, to be taken two to three times a day. Manufactured by Schwabe of Germany, Laitan can be ordered from Victoria Pharmacy Zurich, in Zurich, Switzerland, via e-mail (victoriaapotheke@access.ch).

Other kava products on the European market are formulated with various herbs. Kaviase, for example, is a kava formulation manufactured by Merrell Dow for the French market. Kaviase, used to treat urinary infections, contains the diuretic herb uva ursi and a urinary antiseptic called methenamine.

Potters Herbal Supplies of Great Britain manufactures two kava products: Antiglan, containing saw palmetto extract, kava, equisetum, and hydrangea, for bladder discomfort; and Protat, with cornsilk and kava, also for bladder problems.

Other pharmacological kava preparations available in Europe include Viocava in Switzerland and Mosaro in Austria.

KAVA QUALITY

In the herbal supplement industry today, there are few uniform quality-control standards in place. Raw herbs come from many parts of the world where ideas of cleanliness and purity may be quite different from those in the United States. A related problem is adulteration—substituting one herb for another, or padding the product with a substance not on the label. Supplement suppliers—the people who produce the raw materials used in supplements and sell them to supplement makers—are often guilty of this practice.

Adulteration typically occurs when there is a shortage of an herb coupled with intense consumer demand. To meet the demand, the supplier is tempted to substitute ingredients. This has already occurred with two popular botanicals: St. John's wort, used to treat depression, and saw palmetto, a remedy for a condition called benign prostate enlargement.

In 1997 a laboratory found a St. John's wort sample that was made with an unknown botanical and laced with synthetic hypericin (one of the active ingredients in the herb). In the case of saw palmetto, a poor harvest in 1995 caused a shortage of the herb. To compensate, a vegetable oil was used to replace part of the herb's fatty acids and the product was sold to supplement manufacturers. The real losers in such cases are consumers, who are buying supplements that may not work because they lack the active ingredients to do the job.

A 1981 study reported the adulteration of some Fijian kava powder; however, there have been no recently reported cases. Currently demand for kava is rising so fast that some manufacturers already fear shortages, since the plant usually takes at least two or three years to mature. A shortage could tempt some unscrupulous suppliers to spike their raw materials with the wrong stuff.

Many reputable companies do apply sophisticated quality assurance checks to their products, and these are often noted on the product's label. For example, the kava supplement Kavatrol, made by Natrol, checks purity and potency through "high pressure liquid chromatography." So do many other kava makers. This is a process in which a liquid is separated into its components to check the concentration of active ingredients.

There's more good news on this front: Some twenty-six global botanical companies have already banded together to establish standards for assuring quality and purity of herbal supplements.

Read the labels before you purchase any kava product. Some kava supplements are not manufactured from the roots of the plant and therefore are of inferior quality. Read the label or product information to make sure the supplement is derived from the root, the most potent part of the kava plant.

Also, make sure the label gives

- the amount of kava present in the supplement
- the percentage of kavalactones present (the higher the percentage, the more potent the product)
- full disclosure of any other ingredients
- expiration or best-if-used-by date
- contact information such as phone number, address, or web address
- interactions with other herbs and medicines, as well as cautions for use.

KAVA MAKERS

Here is a partial list of reputable companies currently marketing kava products. In some cases, you can order products directly from the company's Web site.

Better Living Products
801 Lane Street
Irving, TX 75061
972–579–8080
www.betterlivingusa.com

Better Living Products produces micronized kava powder in one- and two-kilogram packages (2.2 pounds per kilogram). Sample recipes and mixing instructions are included with each order. You order the product by calling 972–579–8080. The company accepts Discover/Novus, Visa, and MasterCard.

Elixr Tonics & Teas
8612 Melrose Avenue
Los Angeles, CA 90069
888–4TONICS
Fax: 310–657–9311
www.elixirnet.com

Elixr Tonics & Teas, a popular stopping-off point in southern California, is known for its refreshing and therapeutic concoctions. The company has a staff of eight nationally certified, California-state-licensed herbalists on duty seven days a week. Elixr produces all of its own products in affiliated, internationally inspected laboratories, according to strict standards. These products are available by mail order, and the company publishes a product catalog. Elixr accepts checks, money orders, MasterCard, Visa, and American Express. You can even request that an Elixr herbalist fax a list of its products and their descriptions to your health care practitioner.

Three kava products are sold, both in single herb and tonic formulations. These include: Kava Calm Tonic (2-oz. liquid), formulated with reishi mushroom and polygala; Kava Kava (single herb, liquid, or capsule), made from kava root grown in Vanuatu; and Valerian Slumber Tonic Formula (2-oz. liquid), made with the herbs kava, valerian, polygala, zizyphus, and passion-flower. (See appendix B for an Elixr tonic recipe submitted by the company's herbalists.)

Enzymatic Therapy
825 Challenger Drive
Green Bay, WI 54311
1–920–469–1313
www.enzy.com

An FDA-registered manufacturer, Enzymatic Therapy manufactures and distributes more than two hundred natural medicines, nutritional supplements, vitamins, and herbal extracts. It was the first company in the United States to introduce the natural arthritis remedy, glucosamine sulfate, and the memory enhancer, ginkgo biloba, among other supplements. You can purchase Enzymatic Therapy products in health food stores.

The company has a research team headed up by Michael Murray, N.D., a well-respected naturopath physician and author. The company also works with Lehning Laboratories of Metz, France, a highly regarded homeopathic firm in Europe.

One of Enzymatic Therapy's premier kava products is Kava-55, the only kava product recommended by Harold

Bloomfield, M.D., in his book *Healing Anxiety with Herbs*. The product contains 150 milligrams of kava extract per capsule and is standardized for 55 percent kavalactones. It delivers 82.5 milligrams of kavalactones per softgel. The company also makes Kava-30, with 250 milligrams of kava root extract in each capsule, standardized to contain 30 percent kavalactones and delivering 75 milligrams of kavalactones; KavaTone, which contains kava and vitamins; and St. John's wort, which is a formulation of St. John's wort, kava, and valerian.

Kava Kauai
P.O. Box 1202
Kapaa, HI 96746
1–800–626–0883
www.kauaisource.com

Kava Kauai imports Fijian kava root grown on the island of Vanua Levu, known for its potent strains of kava. The company's kava is 100 percent *waka*, a top grade. It is made from the lateral roots, which supposedly contain the highest concentration of kavalactones.

Kava Kauai makes four products: Waka Grade Kava Root in $1/2$- or 1-pound quantities; Bee Mellow, a blend of pure Hawaiian honey and sifted kava-root powder; Buzz Honey, a multiherb formulation containing pure Hawaiian honey, guarana, kava, ginkgo biloba extract, bee pollen, and licorice root; and Double Root Extract, a concentrated alcohol extract of kava. You can purchase any of these products from the company's Web site and pay for your order by credit card. Kava Kauai accepts MasterCard, Visa, and American Express. The company's Web site has an order form that you can print out, and submit by fax (1–800–626–0883). Or you can order by phone by calling 1–800–626–0883 (United States orders), or 1–808–821–1039 (for orders outside the United States).

Kava King
P.O. Box 721
Ormond Beach, FL 32175
Kava Hot Line: 1–800–638–0082
www.kavaking.com

Kava King makes two excellent kava products, both ground from the dried root of the plant. One of these products is a "ready-to-use" form, which means you can mix it directly in water (no straining required). This product comes in three flavors: traditional banana/vanilla; plain, naturally flavored; and cocoa flavored. It provides 500 milligrams of kavalactones. The other product, which provides 200 milligrams of kavalactones per serving, requires mixing with water and filtering through a mesh cloth. You can order online and pay for your kava with Visa or MasterCard.

Madis Botanicals
375 Huyler Street
South Hackensack, NJ 07606
Phone: 201–440–5000
Fax: 201–342–8000
www.pureworld.com

Founded in 1959, Madis Botanicals is a leading worldwide manufacturer of botanical extracts and today operates one of the largest extraction facilities in North

America. The company produces and sells solid, fluid, and powdered extracts, is an FDA-registered manufacturer, and serves companies in the food, beverage, nutraceutical, and cosmetic industries.

Madis Botanicals produces a variety of kava products, and these include KavaPure Kava SG 70 milligrams, a softgel capsule with 70 milligrams kavalactones per capsule; KavaPure Kava PE 40%, a powdered extract with 40 percent kavalactones; KavaPure Kava PE 30%, a powdered extract with 30 percent kavalactones; and KavaPure Kava FE, a fluid extract with 150 milligrams kavalactones.

The company's Web site contains excellent product data, along with comprehensive information on kava.

Natrol, Inc.
Chatsworth, CA 91311
1–818–739–6000
www.natrol.com

Natrol is a leading supplement company that was founded in 1980 as a small cosmetics business. It launched its first dietary supplement in 1982 and today manufactures Kavatrol, a well-known kava supplement available in capsules and softgels. Other major products include those formulated with ginkgo biloba, melatonin, DHEA, and St. John's wort.

The company has an extensive product line of vitamins, minerals, herbs, specialty formulas, and diet aids. Products bearing the Natrol name are sold in health food stores, pharmacies, supermarkets, and even in hotels and airports, in the United States and in many countries throughout the world.

Nature's Way
Springville, UT 84663
1–801–489–1520
www.naturesway.com

One of the country's largest and most respected manufacturers, Nature's Way had a near miraculous founding.
Seeking a way to relieve the suffering of his gravely ill
wife, founder Tom Murdock discovered the healing benefits of chaparral, a shrubby plant that grows in the South-
west. Remarkably, his wife recovered after being treated
with chaparral. In response, Murdock founded Nature's
Way Research Laboratories in 1969 to market chaparral
tablets.

   Nature's Way grew steadily over the years, and today
offers more than 350 products, from herbs to vitamins
and minerals. Among these products is Kava Kava Root,
which contains 425 milligrams of kava per capsule. Nature's Way supplements are sold in health food stores
throughout the United States.

Solgar
Technical Services Department
500 Willow Tree Road
Leonia, NJ 07605
1–201–944–2311
www.solgar.com

Founded in 1947 Solgar produces and markets an extensive line of nutritional supplements. The company developed the first capsules made entirely from all-vegetable
sources. In 1978 Solgar established the Solgar Nutritional
Research Center, the first of its kind in the supplement

industry, to pioneer and sponsor studies on nutritional supplements.

Solgar manufactures Full Potency Kava Kava Root Vegicaps, which contain 150 milligrams of standardized kava kava root extract (30% kavalactones); and 150 milligrams of raw kava kava root powder. Solgar products are sold in health food stores nationwide.

THE NATURAL MEDICINE PROMISE OF KAVA

Clearly, it is as a natural plant medicine that kava holds its greatest promise. In fact, it is well on its way to becoming one of the top plant medicines of the twenty-first century. It's a virtually safe, natural, nonaddictive substance that when taken in moderate amounts for a short time has the power to calm your body and mind, promote restful sleep, banish a bad mood, relax muscular tension and spasms, and soothe anxiety. Use it wisely, and you won't be disappointed.

Appendix A

KAVA QUESTIONS AND ANSWERS

WHY HAVEN'T MORE STUDIES ON KAVA BEEN DONE IN THE UNITED STATES?

It's true that most kava research has been conducted in Germany and other European nations where herbal medicine is more accepted and widespread. One of the most significant studies ever conducted on kava was done recently in the United States. Researchers at Virginia Commonwealth University found that kava significantly reduced everyday stress in people who used it for four weeks. Kavatrol was the supplement used. To date, the research on kava is promising, and we're likely to see more studies conducted in the United States.

I JUST CAN'T STAND THE TASTE OF KAVA. ISN'T THERE A BETTER WAY TO TAKE IT?

There is little you can do to mask the strong, earthy taste of dried root kava. Your best bet is to take the capsules and follow the manufacturer's recommended dosage.

CAN KAVA HELP ME LOSE WEIGHT?

Kava is believed to be thermogenic; that is, it may raise body temperature and thus burn additional calories. The herb has been used in some parts of the world as a weight-loss agent. But proof of this is very sketchy.

However, you might consider supplementing with kava if you eat when stressed out or down in the dumps. Emotional eating is a habit that can pile on the pounds unless you get it under control. Kava just might be a way to iron out the stress while you curb your overeating.

Also, kava (particularly a cold infusion of dried root) may suppress your appetite—an effect that was noticed as early as 1908 by scientists visiting the islands of Oceania.

DOES KAVA CAUSE ANY ALLERGIES?

Kava is a member of the pepper plant family, so if you're allergic to pepper, avoid supplementing with kava.

AFTER TAKING KAVA, I DIDN'T REALLY SLEEP THAT WELL. ISN'T KAVA SUPPOSED TO HELP YOU SLEEP BETTER?

In most cases, yes. However, everyone reacts to supplements and drugs quite differently. If you suffer from insomnia, give kava a second chance. It may be that your body just needs to get used to it. If you still have trouble sleeping, discontinue the kava.

HOW LONG DOES IT TAKE KAVA TO WORK?

Generally, kava is quite rapid-acting. If you supplement with the dried root powder, you may feel its effects within fifteen to thirty minutes. The capsules may act more slowly, although there may not be any noticeable effect. The capsules slowly regulate your system behind the scenes to decrease stress.

Kava is absorbed faster when taken with a little oil or fat. That's because kavalactones are lipid soluble (they dissolve in fat).

The various kavalactones are absorbed at different rates, too. Kavain and dihydrokavain, for example, enter the brain more easily than do other kavalactones.

WILL KAVA MAKE ME MORE CREATIVE?

It's hard to say for sure, but it might. Vincent Lebot in *Kava: The Pacific Elixir* says that songwriters on Vanuatu, when hired to compose songs, start the creative process by retreating to forests believed to be inhabited by their ancestral spirits. The songwriter sits in the forest and drinks his kava. He listens intently, in hopes of hearing an ancestor sing a song that he can then learn and teach to others.

IF KAVA IS APPROVED AS A DIETARY SUPPLEMENT, DOES IT HAVE ANY NUTRITIONAL VALUE?

Yes. According to analyses by geneticist Vincent Lebot, dried kava rootstock is 43 percent carbohydrate, 20 percent fiber, 12 percent water, 3.6 percent protein, and 3.2 percent minerals (mostly potassium). Kavalactones make up 15 percent of the rootstock. They are found in the fat-soluble resin of the root.

However, you should not look to kava as a source of nutrients. A well-balanced diet of food provides those.

I'M AFRAID TO TELL MY DOCTOR I'M TAKING KAVA. I'M NOT SURE HE'LL UNDERSTAND.

Many doctors vary widely in their opinions of herbal products. And, according to research, less than a third of patients tell their physicians they are using alternative therapies. However, it is critical that you inform your doctor of your decision to take kava. Herbs—including kava—can interact in negative ways with prescription drugs, or cause reactions that are hard to pin down medically, unless your doctor knows what you're taking. If your doctor asks you what medications you're taking or if anything has changed since your last visit, simply tell him or her you're using kava. You may want to send your doctor research and literature on the herb, too.

I'M TAKING QUITE A FEW PRESCRIPTION MEDICATIONS. WILL KAVA INTERACT NEGATIVELY WITH THESE DRUGS?

Kava should not be taken if you're currently taking a sedative, antianxiety drug, tranquilizer, or antidepressant. Nor should it be used in conjunction with antihistamines. Kava could counteract or interfere with the action of other drugs. To be on the safe side, it is probably not a good idea for you to use kava while under medication. Be sure to confirm this with your physician, however.

KAVA ISN'T ADDICTING, BUT CAN'T IT BE HABIT-FORMING?

Yes. Any behavior, positive or negative, can become a habit, and kava drinking is no exception. You can see this in the Aboriginal communities where people go on kava-drinking binges for days at a time. Addiction, on the other hand, implies a physiological dependency. Kava is not known to produce such a dependency.

CAN KAVA BE DETECTED IN DRUG TESTS?

According to Ray Sahelian, M.D., writing in *Kava: The Miracle Antianxiety* herb, kava can be detected in drug tests but only if you request that the testing laboratory analyze your urine for the presence of kava metabolites.

WILL MY PHARMACIST BE FAMILIAR WITH KAVA?

Probably. Many pharmacists are well acquainted with herbs and their medicinal uses. At least one major drug-store chain, Rite Aid, regularly trains its pharmacists on supplements and herbs to keep them up to date on developments in the health food industry.

WHAT IS THE BEST WAY TO TAKE KAVA?

There really is no best way. Most people, however, literally can't stomach the taste of the dried kava powder mixed with water. Some of the mixable dried powders are fairly strong and may cause nausea. In this case, capsules would be preferable. Capsules are also more convenient because they require no mixing or straining. Kava extracts are a convenient option, too.

IF I TAKE KAVA PILLS, WILL THEY MAKE ME FEEL "ZONED-OUT" AT WORK?

No—the latest research indicates that kava capsules taken in recommended doses of 60 to 120 milligrams of kava-lactones a day have no reported negative effect on mental or motor skills. In fact, kava may make you more alert mentally. It works slowly behind the scenes to regulate your system. Just don't overdose on the capsules. Take them for no longer than three months.

Worth mentioning, too, is an experiment that was conducted in 1958 in which researchers looked into what effect large doses of kava had on human volunteers. Over a two-hour period, the volunteers were given six pints of a kava infusion (that's a lot of kava). Afterward, they looked sleepy, and their eyes were a little bloodshot and watery. Their pupils were enlarged and reacting slowly to light. Speech was barely affected. Additionally, the volunteers could walk a straight line and run up stairs two at a time.

CAN CHILDREN TAKE KAVA?

There is no research supporting the use of kava in children. Until studies are conducted, it may be neither wise nor safe to give your children kava. Children under stress or suffering from anxiety should be treated with nondrug, behavioral approaches first, before they are given medication. But if you are considering any form of herbal therapy for your child, consult your pediatrician first.

SHOULD I TAKE MY KAVA CAPSULES AT THE SAME TIME AS I TAKE MY REGULAR NUTRITIONAL SUPPLEMENTS?

Generally, kava supplements should be taken between meals on an empty stomach for better uptake by the body. Your vitamins, minerals, and other nutritional supplements should be taken with meals. They are absorbed better when consumed with food.

WILL RELIGIOUS GROUPS BE AGAINST THE USE OF KAVA?

In the 1800s, when missionaries went to the South Pacific islands, they were initially against kava and wiped it out in some areas. Today, however, this opposition has largely faded. In fact, many denominations on the islands incorporate kava into their worship services and promote kava drinking over alcohol consumption.

Kava—like anything in this world—is abusable. This is evident in the Aboriginal communities in Australia, where overconsumption of kava has become a real problem in society. What is abused or enslaving (addictive or habit-forming) is usually considered a sin.

Are kava, tranquilizers, and antidepressants a shortcut to happiness that bypasses the character-building discipline of faith and religious belief? This is a question each person has to sort out individually, and perhaps with guidance from the clergy. If you are using a lot of kava or another psychiatric drug on a regular basis to avoid dealing with life issues, then you are probably not using it for the right reasons.

Kava's value is as an herb, not as a recreational drug-like substance. On an Internet chat forum, I read one account of a Christian suffering from panic attacks who was prescribed kava by his doctor. The sufferer began feeling better as a result and counted kava as a part of his spiritual renewal.

Thus, kava can do real good in helping people cope with stress, anxiety, and depression—all of which can be life threatening. Most religions have no problem with using prescription medications and other therapies to facilitate a return to normal mental health.

I'VE SEEN KAVA FORMULATED WITH ST. JOHN'S WORT AND SOLD IN HEALTH FOOD STORES. IS A COMBINATION PRODUCT BETTER THAN KAVA OR ST. JOHN'S WORT ALONE?

Some psychiatrists who prescribe herbal tranquilizers believe strongly that St. John's wort combined with kava is effective in the majority of cases in which patients are suffering from mild to moderate anxiety. To date, however, there has been no research on the effects of combin-

ing the two herbs to treat mental disorders. That doesn't
mean the combination doesn't work, though.

SOME COMPANIES ARE SELLING MELATONIN SUPPLEMENTS FORMULATED WITH KAVA. WHAT IS THE VALUE OF SUCH A PRODUCT?

Melatonin is a natural substance made by the pineal
gland, located in the middle of the brain. Discovered in
1958, melatonin is today available as a supplement, produced synthetically or from animal sources. As many as
20 million consumers use melatonin, spending roughly
$350 million dollars on the supplement annually.

Melatonin's job is to set and regulate the internal
clock that controls the body's natural rhythms. It is
touted as a curative for sleep disorders, an antioxidant
that protects cellular health, and a youth restorer. But
with the exception of sleep experiments, most of the melatonin research has been done with animals. Whether or
not melatonin is the fountain of youth we seek remains to
be seen. Even much of the sleep research is inconclusive.
Melatonin appears to help about one half to two thirds of
the people who take it for sleep. Also, melatonin has
some untoward side effects, including next-day groggi-
ness and aggravation of depression. Make sure to purchase
melatonin made by a reputable manufacturer. Many
brands contain impurities and tiny amounts of the actual
hormone, according to researchers.

Some supplement manufacturers are combining melatonin with kava to create a natural, non-habit-forming
sleep inducer. Separately, both melatonin and kava may
help you sleep better at night. Together, they may restore
a good night's sleep, too, although no research has yet
been conducted on the effectiveness of a kava-melatonin
combo.

WHAT ABOUT GINSENG? IN HEALTH FOOD STORES, I'VE SEEN KAVA SUPPLEMENTS THAT CONTAIN GINSENG.

Ginseng is an herb that comes in three varieties: Asian *(Panax ginseng)*; American *(Panax quinquefolius)*; and Siberian *(Eleutherococcus senticosus)*, which originates from a different species than the Panax classifications. Siberian ginseng is not a true ginseng, but rather a botanical cousin.

Generally safe, ginseng is categorized as an "adaptogen," meaning an agent that helps your body cope with the harmful physical effects of stress. For this reason, it is often combined with kava. Theoretically, ginseng alleviates the physical stress; kava, the mental stress. There's little information on whether this combination works, however. I have read one account in which a woman took a kava/ginseng formula, did well for a couple of weeks, but then began suffering from insomnia and some anxiety. Once she stopped taking the supplement, the symptoms gradually subsided. Mixing various herbal supplements should be approached cautiously.

CAN KAVA BE GROWN IN THE UNITED STATES?

Kava grows in the state of Hawaii and in American Samoa, a U.S. territory. But it cannot grow in the continental United States because it requires a tropical climate, organically rich soil, and lots of rain to thrive.

WHEN I GO TO THE HEALTH FOOD STORE TO BUY KAVA OR ANOTHER HERB, HOW DO I KNOW I'M GETTING WHAT THE PRODUCT CLAIMS TO BE?

At present there are few controls over what goes into supplements, or whether products are even as pure as they should be. That's because herbs are considered food additives, not drugs, and they are therefore not under the same scrutiny by the FDA as drugs. My recommendation is that you purchase kava and other herbal products from reputable companies that have been in the supplement business for a long time. For a list of recommended companies, see chapter 15.

Quality standards in the herbal-products industry are improving. The United States Pharmacopoeia (USP), a body of experts that sets standards for prescription and over-the-counter drugs, is developing guidelines for the manufacturers of herbal products. In the future any herbal product that carries the USP designation will be obligated voluntarily to meet USP criteria for quality, strength, purity, and packaging. This move will certainly give consumers piece of mind that a product conforms to certain minimum standards.

Appendix B

KAVA COOKING

The following three recipes are printed with the permission of Better Living Products, Processor, Wholesaler, and Retailer of Kava Root Products, 801 Lane Street, Irving, Texas, 75061, 972–579–8080. www.betterlivingusa.com.

The Kava Party Recipe
1 two-liter bottle 7-Up or lemon-lime soda
4 tablespoons lime juice
8 tablespoons Better Living Micronized Kava Powder
Sweeten to taste

Mix in a large bowl to allow room for soda to foam. Stir frequently to prevent settling.

Kava Espresso

Kava espresso, or low liquid method, is for individual use, for quickly winding down from a stressful day. Put one or two tablespoons of Better Living Micronized Kava powder in a cup and add $1/4$ to $1/2$ cup water, 1 tablespoon lime juice, and 1 packet sweetener. Stir until smooth; adjust water to desired consistency. As an alternative to lime juice, try equal amounts kava powder and Tang in $1/2$ cup water. (Suggestion: Try one tablespoon of kava first.)

Warm Kava Tea

For a warm, relaxing drink, try one tablespoon Better Living Micronized powder in warm (not hot) double strength coffee, tea, or hot chocolate. Use decaffeinated varieties to promote a more restful sleep.

The following recipe and product information are printed with the permission of Elixr Tonics & Teas, 8612 Melrose Avenue, Los Angeles, CA 90069, 888–4TONICS, Fax: 310–657–9311, www.elixirnet.com.

*Kava Pacifica

2 droppers Kava Calm Tonic
2 droppers Flowing Energy Tonic
1 dropper Guarana Seed Extract

Combine with 8 to 10 ounces juice or your favorite tea and honey.

Product information: Kava Calm Tonic is an Elixr product based on kava, reishi mushroom, and polygala root to help generally calm and smooth away stress.

($22.00 for a 2-oz. concentrated extract); Flowing Energy Tonic is a Chinese herb-based formula containing bupleurum, cyperus, and licorice root. ($24.00 for 2-oz. concentrated extract); Guarana seed contains guaranine, a safe caffeinelike constituent that keeps the drink from becoming too sedating. ($13.00 for 1-oz. concentrated extract)

Elixr sells these and other kava-based products on its Web site (www.elixirnet.com), through mail order at 888–4TONICS, and from selected retailers. A product catalog is available upon request.

ADDITIONAL RECIPES

Kava Cappuccino Frappe

2 tablespoons cocoa-flavored kava powder
$1/2$ cup chilled coffee
$1/2$ cup skim milk
2 heaping teaspoons sugar (or to taste)
$1/8$ teaspoon cinnamon (or to taste)
3-4 ice cubes

Place all ingredients in a blender and blend until smooth. Makes 1 to 2 servings.

Tropical Kava

1 cup tropical fruit juice such as a peach/mango/orange product, or apple juice
2 tablespoons ready-to-use kava powder

Place all ingredients in a blender and blend until smooth.

Appendix C

KAVA IN CYBERSPACE

If you would like to find out more about kava, the World Wide Web is loaded with it! Simply type the keyword "kava" into any search engine, and you'll be bombarded with sites—thousands, to be exact. Most of these sites are selling kava products, however. The Web addresses of the more well-established and reputable kava supplement manufacturers are provided in chapter 14, and they're worth a visit.

To help you navigate through this fray, here are a number of other recommended sites that may be of interest.

Lee Kagan's Kava Page: www.prairienet.org/kagan/kavabib. html#bibliography—This site is an extensive compilation of reference sources for kava, from periodical articles to books to newsgroups.

Hawaii Pacific Index: www.auckland.acnz/lbr/hawjourn.htm —Here you can examine holdings from the University of Hawaii at Manoa and other libraries. Nonstudent, nonfaculty visitors can set up an account to order articles from certain indexes. Payable by credit card, this feature is a fax-on-demand service, and the articles are faxed to you within moments of ordering.

Deja News, Inc.: www.dejanews.com—By searching the site's database for "kava," you can read comments from people who have tried the herb.

Medline: www.ncbi.nlm.nih.gov—This link from the National Library of Medicine provides abstracts on the many scientific studies conducted on kava. Simply type in "kava" under the word search option, and numerous abstracts will appear.

Pacific Forum: www.pacificforum.com—This site gives you access to the "Kava Bowl," in which people discuss kava and other Pacific issues in newsgroups and chat rooms.

Electronic Library: www.elibrary.com—For news articles on kava, this site is a good source. It's a subscription service, however, payable by credit card. Simply type in the keyword "kava," and elibrary will pull up all available stories on kava.

Herb Research Foundation: www.herbs.org—This organization offers extensive information on herbs and their uses.

Appendix D

KAVA-SPEAK

Aibo: A Fijian term for the strainer used to prepare kava.

'Apu 'ava: A Hawaiian term for the coconut shell in which kava is served.

Bilo ni yagona: A Fijian term for the coconut shell in which kava is served.

Dauvagunu: A Fijian spiritual leader. The literal translation of the word is "an expert at drinking kava."

Grog: A Fijian term for kava.

Ipu 'ava: A Samoan term for the coconut shell in which kava is served.

Kanikana: The Fijian term for a scaly skin condition that afflicts natives who are heavy drinkers of kava (up to half a dozen liters or more a day).

Kanoa: The Hawaiian term for kava bowl.

Maca: A response made by people in a kava circle after you have drunk your kava (Fiji). Translated, *maca* means "it [your bowl] is dry."

Manuia: Means "good luck" in Samoan, should be expressed before drinking kava in a traditional Samoan kava ceremony.

Meke: A party held on Pacific islands for tourists and locals that features kava drinking, traditional food, music, and dancing.

Nahunu: A term used on Vanuatu referring to food that is eaten after you drink kava.

Nakamal: Literally "men's house," kava bars.

Nasara: An open area surrounded by huge banyan trees (on Tanna) where village men gather each evening to drink kava at the *nakamal.*

Nivhau: A Vanuatu kava strainer made from a banana stem.

Sakau: The name given to the kava grown on the island of Pohnpei.

Talanoa: Fijian for "conversation," "chat."

Tanoa: The wooden bowl used in Fiji to mix pulverized kava root with water.

Tau tava: A Samoan term for the strainer used to prepare kava.

Tou'a: The woman who mixes the kava in informal kava circles.

Yagona: Another name for kava in Fiji. Also spelled yanggona.

Yimwayim: A circular area usually shaded by banyan trees where kava ceremonies are held.

References

CHAPTER ONE
The Wonder Herb of the South Pacific

Dentali, S. J. 1997. *Herb safety review: Kava.* Boulder, Colo.: Herb Research Foundation.

Editor. 1997. Kava, the feel-good herb. *Drug Store News* 19: CP17–CP19.

Fackelman, K. A. 1992. Pacific cocktail. *Science News.* June 27:424–25.

Goldberg, B. 1998. Don't be a friendly-fire casualty in the war on disease. *Alternative Medicine.* September: 10–11.

Hendler, S. S. 1992. Tapping the healing power of herbs. *Executive Health's Good Health Report* 28: 1–4.

Hobbs, C. 1991. Adaptogens: All-purpose herbs. *East West* 21: 54–61.

Hocart, C. H., B. Fankhauser, and David W. Buckle. 1993. Chemical archaeology of kava, a potent brew. *Rapid Communications in Mass Spectrometry* 7: 219–24.

Kilham, C. 1998. Kava: a review. Internet Web site: www.pureworld.com/science/kava—review.html.

Miller R. A. 1983. *The Magical and Ritual Use of Herbs.* Rochester, Vt.: Destiny Books.

Natrol. 1996. Kava white paper. Chatsworth, Calif.: Natrol, Inc.

Petersen, A. 1998. The making of an herbal superstar. *The Wall Street Journal.* February (reprint), Princeton, New Jersey: Journal/ Reprints).

Singh, Y. N. 1992. Kava: an overview. *Journal of Ethnopharmacology* 37: 13–45.

Tyler, V. E. 1997. Nature's stress buster. *Prevention. October:* 90– 93.

CHAPTER TWO
Kava Lore

Andersen, J. C. 1995. *Myths and legends of the Polynesians.* Toronto: General Publishing Company.

Bourne, W. 1995. The gospel according to Frum. *Harper's Magazine.* January: 60–68.

Brunton, R. 1989. *The Abandoned Narcotic.* New York: Cambridge University Press.

Dentali, S. J. 1997. *Herb safety review: Kava.* Boulder, Colo.: Herb Research Foundation.

Dolby, V. 1996. Kava: a Polynesian gift for anxiety, tension, and insomnia. *Better Nutrition.* June: 26.

Forster, J. G. A. 1777. *A voyage round the world in his Britannic majesty's sloop* Resolution. London: Hakluyt Society. Quoted in Lebot, *Kava: The Pacific Elixir.*

Guerreiro, A. 1997. The Pacific: The coming of the ancestors. *UNESCO Courier.* December: 14–16.

Kilham, C. 1996. *Kava: Medicine Hunting in Paradise.* Rochester, Vt.: Park Street Press.

Lebot, V., M. Merlin, and L. Lindstrom. 1997. *Kava: The Pacific Elixir.* New Haven: Yale University Press.

Long, J. D. 1998. Pacific: Decline and fall of world religions, 1900–2025. Global Evangelization Movement Web site, www.gem-werc.org.

Luders, D. 1996. Legend and history: Did the Vanuatu-Tonga trade cease in A.D. 1447? *The Journal of the Polynesian Society* 105: 287–310.

Lynch, J. 1996. Kava-drinking in southern Vanuatu: Melanesian drinkers, Polynesian roots. *The Journal of the Polynesian Society* 105: 27–40.

Miller R. A. 1983. *The Magical and Ritual Use of Herbs.* Rochester, Vt.: Destiny Books.

Price, A. G., ed. 1971. *The Explorations of Captain James Cook in the Pacific as Told by Selections of His Own Journals 1768–1779.* New York: Dover Publications, Inc.

Singh, Y. N. 1992. Kava: An overview. *Journal of Ethnopharmacology* 37: 13–45.

Singh, Y. N., and M. Blumenthal. 1998. Kava culture, then and now. *Herbs for Health,* January/February, Internet edition (www.aznet.net/~benhess/kavac.html).

Visser, E. P. 1994. Skeletal evidence of kava use in prehistoric Fiji. *The Journal of the Polynesian Society* 103: 299–317.

Von Bibra, E. 1995. *Plant Intoxicants.* Rochester, Vt.: Healing Arts Press.

Whistler, W. A. 1992. *Tongan herbal medicine.* Honolulu, Hawaii: Isle Botanica.

CHAPTER THREE
Kava, Kava, Everywhere

Brevoort, B. 1996. The medicinal and spiritual properties of kava. *Nutrition Science News,* April. Internet Web site: www.delicious-online.com/health/articles.

Brunton, R. 1989. *The Abandoned Narcotic.* New York: Cambridge University Press.

Editor. 1998. Kava lounge. Internet Web site: newyork. citysearch.com.

Fackelman, K. A. 1992. Pacific cocktail. *Science News.* June 27: 424–25.

Gomes, A. 1998. Big Isle eyes $12 million market for medicinal plants. *Pacific Business News.* January 19.

Goodwin, B. 1998. *Frommer's South Pacific.* New York: Macmillan.

Hocart, C. H., B. Fankhauser, and David W. Buckle. 1993. Chemical archaeology of kava, a potent brew. *Rapid Communications in Mass Spectrometry* 7: 219–24.

Lebot, V., M. Merlin, and L. Lindstrom. 1997. *Kava: The Pacific Elixir.* New Haven: Yale University Press.

Lindstrom, L. 1991. Kava, cash, and custom in Vanuatu. *CS Quarterly* 15: 28–31.

Miller R. A. 1983. *The Magical and Ritual Use of Herbs.* Rochester, Vt.: Destiny Books.

Parker, J. 1997. Health hut's kava-kava shot competes against java java. *The Miami Student Outline.* April 18: 1.

Pettera, A. 1997. Restaurant notes. *Los Angeles Times.* July 31: 41.

Pradash, N., J. F. Brown, and Y. Wang. 1994. An embryological study of kava, *piper methysticum. Australian Journal of Botany* 42: 231–37.

Shadbolt, M. and O. Ruhen. 1968. *Isles of the South Pacific.* Washington, D.C.: National Geographic Society.

Singh, Y. N. 1992. Kava: an overview. *Journal of Ethnopharmacology* 37: 13–45.

Singh, Y. N. and M. Blumenthal. 1998. Kava culture, then and now. *Herbs for Health,* January/February, Internet Web site: www.aznet.net/~benhess/kavac.html.

Stanley, D. 1996. 6th ed. *South Pacific Handbook.* Chico, Calif.: Moon Publications, Inc.

Withey, L. 1987. *Voyages of Discovery: Captain Cook and the Exploration of the Pacific.* Los Angeles: University of California Press.

CHAPTER FOUR
Kava Experiences

Leeds, J. and P. Levikow. 1997. Man whose drink made revelers ill enters guilty pleas. *Los Angeles Times.* November 4:3.

Mathews, J. D., M. D. Riley, L. Fejo, et al. 1988. Effects of the heavy usage of kava on physical health: Summary of a pilot survey in an aboriginal community. *Medical Journal of Australia* 148: 548–55.

Natrol, Inc. 1998. "I love this stuff," says Kavatrol study participant. Natrol press release, April 4.

Newsgroups/Web sites sampled include: www.dejanews.com; www.hyperreal.com; www.pacificforum.com; and www.lycaeum. org.

Pacific Islands Development Program. 1998. Kiribati kava drinking affecting family health and welfare. *Pacific Islands Report.* March 16.

Pappas, B. 1997. Transparent eyeball. *Forbes Magazine.* December 12:39.

Singh, Y. N. 1992. Kava: An overview. *Journal of Ethnopharmacology* 37: 13–45. Quoting Torrey, W. 1848. *Torrey's*

Narrative, or the life and adventures of William Torrey. Boston: A. J. Wright; Emerson, O. P. 1903. The awa habit of the Hawaiians. *Hawaiian Annual,* 130–40; and Lemert, E. M. 1967. Secular use of kava in Tonga. *Quarterly Journal of Studies on Alcohol* 28: 328–41.

Spillane, P., D. A. Fisher, and B. J. Currier. 1997. Neurological manifestations of kava intoxication. *Medical Journal of Australia* 167: 172–73.

CHAPTER FIVE
The Kick That Kava Gives

Agricultural Research Services. 1998. Dr. Duke's Phytochemical and Ethnobotanical Databases. Beltsville, Md.: United States Department of Agriculture.

Argyll Laboratories, 1961. Harvard Letters. *www.leary.com/ archives/text/Letters/Harvard/66frArgyll.html.*

Bower, B. 1997. Brain structure sounds off to fear. *Science News* 151:38.

Caldwell, M. 1994. Brain faces up to fear, social signs. *Science News* 146:406.

———. 1995. Kernel of fear. *Discover.* June: 96–102.

Hocart, C. H., B. Fankhauser, and David W. Buckle. 1993. Chemical archaeology of kava, a potent brew. *Rapid Communications in Mass Spectrometry* 7: 219–24.

Jussofie, A., A. Schmitz, and C. Hiemke. 1994. Kavapyrone-enriched extract from Piper methysticum as modulator of the GABA binding site in different regions of the rat brain. *Psychopharmacology* 116: 469–74.

Kilham, C. 1996. *Kava: Medicine Hunting in Paradise.* Rochester, Vt.: Park Street Press.

———. 1998. Kava, the tranquil plant. *Total Health for Longevity.* April/May: 22–24.

Lebot, V., M. Merlin, and L. Lindstrom. 1997. *Kava: The Pacific Elixir.* New Haven: Yale University Press.

LeDoux, J. E. 1995. Emotion: Clues from the brain. *Annual Review of Psychology* 46: 209–55.

Reuters News Service. 1997. Brain sites for depression symptoms. November 13.

Schelosky, L., Raffaul, C., 1995. Kava and dopamine antagonism. *Journal of Neurology, Neurosurgery, and Psychiatry* 58: 639–40.

Seitz, U., A. Schule, and J. Glietz. 1997. [3H]-monoamine uptake inhibition properties of kava pyrones. *Planta Medica* 63: 548–49.

Singh, Y. N. 1983. Effects of kava on neuromuscular transmission and muscle contractility. *Journal of Ethnopharmacology.* 7: 267–76.

———. 1992. Kava: An overview. *Journal of Ethnopharmacology* 37: 13–45.

Walden, J., J. von Wegerer, U. Winter, M. Berger, and H. Grunze. 1997. Effects of kawain and dihydromethysticin on field potential changes in the hippocampus. *Progress in Neuropsychopharmacology and Biological Psychiatry* 21: 697–706.

Walji, H. 1997. *Kava: Nature's Relaxant for Anxiety, Stress, and Pain.* Prescott, Ariz.: Hohm Press.

CHAPTER SIX
Kava: Nature's Stress Cure

Berardelli, P. 1996. Chronic stress shrinks brains. *Insight on the News.* October 28: 44–45.

Carpi, J. 1996. Stress . . . it's worse than you think. *Psychology Today.* January/February: 34–37.

Dua J., and L. Hargreaves. 1992. Effect of aerobic exercise on negative affect, positive affect, stress, and depression. *Perceptual Motor Skills* 75:355–61.

Farrington, J. 1996. Stress and what you can do about it. *Current Health* 2: 6–11.

Fischman, J. 1987. Type A on trial. *Psychology Today*. February: 42–48.

Ford, N. D. 1992. The heartbreaking news about stress. *Health News & Reviews*. Summer: 7.

Geier, T. 1996. Hotheads and heart attacks. *U.S. News & World Report*. November: 11, 16.

Houck, C. 1996. When stress gets under your skin. *Good Housekeeping*. May: 52–54.

International Society of Sport Psychology Position Statement. 1992. Physical activity and psychological benefits. *The Physician and Sportsmedicine* 20: 179–84.

Langer, S. 1995. Nutritionally coping with stress. *Better Nutrition*. July: 42–44.

Lark, S. N. 1994. Strike back at high anxiety: Natural ways to stay calm in stressful times. *Vegetarian Times*. February: 90–92.

Lohmeier, L. 1992. Stress that strikes you in the stomach. *Current Health 2*. November: 22–23.

Moran, V. 1989. Mind over immunity. *Vegetarian Times*. November: 32–36.

Murray, F. 1992. The healthy approach to stress control. *Better Nutrition*. June: 20–22.

Peltz, P. 1998. The kava craze. American Broadcasting Company *20/20*. June 22.

Petersen, A. 1998. The making of an herbal superstar. *The Wall Street Journal*. February (reprint, Princeton, New Jersey: Journal/ Reprints).

Rapaport, W. S. 1993. He who laughs . . . lasts longer and lives better. *Diabetes in the News*. November/December: 12–14.

Singh, N. N., C. R. Ellis, A. M. Best, et al. 1998. Kavatrol reduces daily stress and anxiety in adults. (unpublished). Chatsworth, Calif.: Natrol, Inc.

CHAPTER SEVEN
Easing Anxiety

Broocks, A., B. Bandelow, G. Pekrun, et al. 1998. Comparison of aerobic exercise, clomipramine, and placebo in the treatment of panic disorder. *American Journal of Psychiatry* 155: 603–09.

Butler, K. 1997. After shock. *Health.* October: 104–09.

Dilsaver, S. C. 1989. Generalized anxiety disorder. *American Family Physician* 39: 137–44.

Kilham, C. 1997. Kava for anxiety and insomnia. *Nutrition Science News.* May. Internet Web site: www.delicious-online.com/health/articles.

Kinzler, E., J. Kromer, and E. Lehmann. 1991. Effect of a special kava extract in patients with anxiety, tension, and excitation states of a non-psychotic genesis. Double blind study with placebos over four weeks. *Arzneimittel-Forschung* 41: 584–88.

Larson, D. E., ed. 1990. *Mayo Clinic Family Health Book.* New York: William Morrow and Company, Inc.

Medical Economics Data. 1993. *The PDR family guide to prescription drugs.* Montvale, N.J.: Medical Economics Data, Inc.

Reichert, R. G. 1997. *Kava Kava: The Anti-anxiety Herb that Relaxes and Sharpens the Mind.* New Canaan, Conn.: Keats Publishing, Inc.

Volz, H. P., and M. Kieser. 1997. Kava-kava extract WS 1490 versus placebo in anxiety disorders—a randomized placebo-controlled 25-week outpatient trial. *Pharmacopsychiatry* 30: 1–5.

Walley, E. J., D. K. Beebe, and J. L. Clark, 1994. Management of common anxiety disorders. *American Family Physician* 50: 1745–55.

Warnecke, G. 1991. Psychosomatic dysfunctions in the female climacteric. Clinical effectiveness and tolerance of kava extract WS 1490. *Fortschritte der Medizin* 109: 119–22.

CHAPTER EIGHT
Beating the Blues

Bower, B. 1994. Stress may take two paths in depression. *Science News* 146:52.

Colchamiro, R. 1998. Worting away depression. *American Druggist.* January: 28–31.

Editor. 1997. Depression linked to fracture risk. *USA Today.* October: 6.

Grewal, H. 1992. Women's health: Biochemical depression. *Total Health,* 27–29.

Hippisley-Cox, J., K. Fielding, and M. Pringle. 1998. Depression as a risk factor for ischaemic heart disease in men: Population-based case-control study. *British Medical Journal* 316: 1714–19.

Larson, D. E., ed. 1990. *Mayo Clinic Family Health Book.* New York: William Morrow and Company, Inc.

Maynard, R. 1997. An invisible killer. *Chatelaine.* March: 8.

McCann, L., and D. S. Holmes. 1984. Influence of aerobic exercise on depression. *Journal of Personality and Social Psychology* 46: 1142–47.

McCord, H. 1998. Improve your mood with food. *Prevention.* August: 57.

Medical Economics Data. 1993. *The PDR family guide to prescription drugs.* Montvale, N.J.: Medical Economics Data, Inc.

Monahan, T. 1986. Exercise and depression: Swapping sweat for serenity? *The Physician and Sportsmedicine* 14:192, 194.

Payer, L., D. Willensky, W. Conkling, and E. Stark. 1991. Quicker fixer uppers. *American Health*: 43–50.

Peltz, P. 1998. The kava craze. American Broadcasting Company *20/20*. June 22.

Shearer, S. L., and G. K. Adams. 1993. Nonpharmacologic aids in the treatment of depression. *American Family Physician* 47: 435–43.

Warnecke, G. 1991. Psychosomatic dysfunctions in the female climacteric. Clinical effectiveness and tolerance of kava extract WS 1490. *Fortschritte der Medizin* 109: 119–22.

Zung, W. W. K., E. Broadhead, and M. E. Roth. 1993. Prevalence of depressive symptoms in primary care. *Journal of Family Practice* 37: 338–44.

CHAPTER NINE
Overcoming Insomnia

Dolby, V. 1998. Fulfill your dreams: Sleep better with natural remedies. *Let's Live*. March: 42–47.

Editor. 1993. Seven keys to the good life. *Tufts University Diet & Nutrition Letter*. August: 1.

Editor. 1996. Why nearly half of all adults have trouble sleeping. *Jet*. January 15: 54–57.

LaForge, R. 1988. Helping the sandman. *Executive Health Report*. May: 8.

Larson, D. E., ed. 1990. *Mayo Clinic Family Health Book*. New York: William Morrow and Company, Inc.

Ludington, A. 1996. Rest: How much is enough? *Vibrant Life*. March/April: 4–6.

Nieman, D. C. 1995. Oh, for a good night's sleep. *Vibrant Life*. July/August: 28–30.

Reichert, R. 1997. *Kava Kava: The Anti-anxiety Herb that Relaxes and Sharpens the Mind.* New Canaan, Conn.: Keats Publishing, Inc.

Toufexis, A. 1990. Drowsy America. *Time.* December 17: 78–84.

White, Linda. 1996. No more tossing and turning: Drug-free ways to get your zzz's. *Vegetarian Times.* November: 34–37.

CHAPTER TEN
More Medical Miracles from Kava

Backhauss, C., and J. Krieglstein. 1992. Extract of kava *(Piper methysticum)* and its methysticin constituents protect brain tissue against ischemic damage in rodents. *European Journal of Pharmacology* 215: 265–69.

Gleitz, J., A. Beile, P. Wilkens, A. Ameri, and T. Peters. 1997. Antithrombotic action of the kava pyrone (+)-kavain prepared from *Piper methysticum* on human platelets. *Plant Medica* 63: 27–30.

Gleitz, J., J. Friese, A. Beile, A. Ameri, and T. Peters. 1996. Anticonvulsive action of (+/−)-kavain estimated from its properties on stimulated synaptosomes and Na+ channel receptor sites. *European Journal of Pharmacology* 315: 89–97.

Jamieson, D. D., and P. H. Duffield. 1990. The antinociceptive actions of kava components in mice. *Clinical Experiments in Pharmacology and Physiology* 17: 495–507.

Johnson, K. 1990. The herbal love potions. *East West.* February: 44–51.

Kleiner, S. M., and M. Greenwood-Robinson. 1998. *Power eating.* Champaign, Ill.: Human Kinetics, Inc.

Kryspin-Exner, K. 1974. The effect of kavain on alcoholic patients in the withdrawal phase. *Muncher/Medizinische/Wochenscrift* 116: 1557–60.

Larson, D. E., ed. 1990. *Mayo Clinic Family Health Book.* New York: William Morrow and Company, Inc.

O'Donnell, S. A. 1998. Can herbs fight cancer? *Prevention.* September: 116–23.

Puotinen, C. J. 1997. Herbs for virility: Natural ways to spruce up your sex appeal. *Vegetarian Times.* May: 80–82.

Reichert, R. 1997. *Kava Kava: The Anti-anxiety Herb that Relaxes and Sharpens the Mind.* New Canaan, Conn.: Keats Publishing, Inc.

Sahelian, R. 1998. *Kava: The Miracle Antianxiety Herb.* New York: St. Martin's Press.

Turner, E. F. 1992. Ask the herbalist. *Nutrition Health Review.* Summer: 16.

Walji, H. 1997. *Kava: Nature's Relaxant for Anxiety, Stress and Pain.* Prescott, Ariz.: Hohm Press.

Williams, G. 1991. Pain! treating and defeating it. *American Health.* November: 45–47.

CHAPTER ELEVEN
Kava versus Prescription Mood Drugs

Alper, J. 1988. Tranquilizers: A user's guide. *Health.* November: 35–40.

Bibeau, T. 1994. The dark side of psychiatric drugs. *USA Today Magazine.* May 1994: 44–47.

Cadieux, R. J. 1996. Azapirones: An alternative to benzodiazepines for anxiety. *American Family Physician* 53: 49–53.

Chollar, S. 1988. Tranquil daze. *Psychology Today.* January: 12.

Danton, W. G., J. Altrocchi, D. Antonuccio, and R. Basta. 1994. Nondrug treatment of anxiety. *American Family Physician* 49: 161–66.

Editor. 1992. Medical update: Are tranquilizers over-prescribed? *Health News.* August: 1.

FDA. 1997. Benzodiazepines and related substances. *Federal Register.* June 19: 33418–24.

Guze, B. H., and M. Gitlin. 1994. New antidepressants and the treatment of depression. *Journal of Family Practice* 38: 49–57.

Lader, M. 1994. Treatment of anxiety. *British Medical Journal* 309: 321–24.

Lindenburg, D., and H. Pitule-Schodel. 1990. D,L-kavain in comparison with oxazepam in anxiety disorders. A double-blind study of clinical effectiveness. *Fortschritte der Medizin* 108: 49–50.

Mauro, J., and P. Breggin. 1994. And Prozac for all. *Psychology Today.* July/August: 44–51.

McBride, G. 1994. America goes crazy for the "happy pill." *British Medical Journal* 308:665.

Medical Economics Data. 1993. *The PDR family guide to prescription drugs.* Montvale, N.J.: Medical Economics Data, Inc.

Munte, T. F., H. J. Heinze, M. Matzke, and J. Steitz. 1993. Effects of oxazepam and an extract of kava roots *(Piper methysticum)* on event-related potentials in a word recognition task. *Neuropsychobiology* 27: 46–53.

Rakel, R. E. 1989. How to use them, what to avoid: Antianxiety agents. *Consultant.* June: 75–80.

Scheller, M. 1997. The brave new world of antidepressants. *Current Health 2.* January: 16–18.

Scripps Howard News Service. Prescription drug pitfalls growing. *Evansville Courier.* 9 June, 1998: A2.

Wagner, J., M. L. Wagner, and W. A. Hening. 1998. Beyond benzodiazepines: Alternative pharmacologic agents for the treatment of insomnia. *Annals of Pharmacotherapy* 32: 680–91.

CHAPTER TWELVE
Kava and Other Calming Herbs

Bergner, P. 1993. Herbs that calm your nerves. *Natural Health.* July/August: 56–58.

Bourin, M., T. Bougerol, B. Guitton, and E. Broutin. 1997. A combination of plant extracts in the treatment of outpatients with adjustment disorder with anxious mood: Controlled study versus placebo. *Fundamentals in Clinical Pharmacologie* 11: 127–32.

Chan, T. Y., C. H. Tang, and J. A. Critchley. 1995. Poisoning due to an over-the-counter hypnotic, Sleep-Qik (hyosine, cyproheptadine, valerian). *Postgraduate Medical Journal* 71: 227–28.

Duke, J. A. 1997. *The green pharmacy.* Emmaus, Penn.: Rodale Press.

Editor. 1995. Aromatherapy: Lavender fragrance is sleep inducing. *The Brown University Long-Term Care Quality Letter.* 16 October: 6.

Editor. 1993. Lavender-oil component shows promise in treating and preventing cancer. *Cancer Research Weekly.* 7 June: 11–12.

Editor. 1995. Lavender scent to treat insomnia. *HealthFacts.* October: 3.

Editor. 1995. Natural cancer-fighter drug is component of oil of lavender. *Cancer Biotechnology Weekly.* 9 October: 7–8.

Editor. 1991. Researchers "discover" herbal sleep remedy. *Nutrition Health Review.* Spring: 7.

FDA. 1997. Benzodiazepines and related substances. *Federal Register.* 19 June: 33418–24.

Finlayson-Dutton, G. 1991. Valerian: Nature's sedative. *East West.* November/December: 50–51.

Foster, S. 1989. Camomile: More than a cup of tea. *Bestways,* 54–55.

————. 1989. Valerian: Europe's sleeping pill. *Bestways.* February: 38–39.

————. 1996. Three top herbs that work so you can sleep. *Better Nutrition.* March: 46–49.

————. 1997. "Perchance to dream . . . ?" Herbs to help us sleep. *Better Nutrition.* March: 64–66.

————. 1997. Phytomedicine—harnessing the healing power of plants: Herbs for the next millennium. *Better Nutrition.* December: 32–35.

Gerhard, U., V. Hobi, R. Kocher, and C. Konig. 1991. Acute sedative effect of an herbal relaxation tablet as compared to that of bromazepam. *Schweizerische Rundschau feur Medizin Praxis* 80: 1481–86.

Gerhard, U., N. Linnenbrink, C. Georghiadou, and V. Hobi. 1996. Viligance-decreasing effects of two plant-derived sedatives. *Schweizerische Rundschau feur Medizin Praxis* 85:473–81.

Goulart, F. S. 1989. How to sleep well without harmful drugs. *Total Health.* December: 37–39.

Griffith, H. W. 1988. *Complete Guide to Vitamins, Minerals & Supplements.* Tucson, Ariz.: Fisher Books.

Harder, P. A. 1998. Self-help strategies for zapping the effects of chronic stress. *Better Nutrition:* 36.

Hien, T. T., and N. J. White. 1993. Quinghaosu. *The Lancet* 341: 603–07.

Hobbs, C. 1990. Get on your nerves: Give your nervous system herbs that can sooth, stimulate or heal. *Vegetarian Times.* July: 73–76.

————. 1992. Cultivate health with herbs. *East West.* September/October: 76–89.

Hochwald, L. 1996. Natural stress solutions. *Natural Health.* May/June: 68–80.

Keville, K. 1990. Chamomile: The soothing herb. *Vegetarian Times.* September: 63–65.

Kort, M. 1997. Natural Rx for depression. *Vegetarian Times.* December: 56–61.

Lee, P. 1990. Valerian. *Total Health.* June: 43–44.

———. 1991. Lemon herbs. *Total Health.* August: 50–52.

McCaleb, R. 1990. Valerian: Nature's potent sleep aid. *Better Nutrition.* August: 20–22.

———. 1991. The soothing effects of chamomile. *Better Nutrition.* May: 24–27.

———. 1993. Chamomile: The world's most soothing herb. *Better Nutrition.* September: 48–50.

———. 1994. Herbal lullabies to gently rock you to sleep. *Better Nutrition.* April: 60–62.

Medina, J. H., V. Haydee, C. Wolfman, et al. 1997. Overview—flavonoids: A new family of benzodiazepine receptor ligands. *Neurachemical Research* 22: 419–25.

Miller, R. A. 1983. *The Magical and Ritual Use of Herbs.* Rochester, Vt.: Destiny Books.

Murray, F. 1996. Menopausal symptoms may respond to the herb, black cohosh. *Better Nutrition.* March: 24.

Natelson, E. J. 1994. Beating stress naturally. *Vegetarian Times.* February: 86–88.

Sakamoto, T., Y. Mitani, and K. Nakajima. 1992. Psychotropic effects of Japanese valerian root extract. *Chemical and Pharmaceutical Bulletin* 40: 758–61.

Scheer, J. F. 1990. Camomile can be everything from toothache remedy to natural hair dye for blondes. *Better Nutrition.* May: 15–17.

———. 1996. Not just for PMS, black cohosh is effective for menopause as well. *Better Nutrition.* April: 32.

Weisbord, S. D., J. B. Soule, and P. L. Kimmel. 1997. Poison on line—acute renal failure caused by oil of wormwood purchased through the Internet. *The New England Journal of Medicine* 337: 825–27.

White, Linda. 1996. No more tossing and turning: Drug-free ways to get your zzz's. *Vegetarian Times*. November: 34–37.

CHAPTER THIRTEEN
Other Natural Tension-Tamers

Abou-Saleh, M. T., and A. Coppen. 1986. The biology of folate in depression: Implications for nutritional hypotheses of the psychoses. *Journal of Psychiatric Research* 20: 91–101.

Banderet, L. E., and H. R. Lieberman. 1989. Treatment with tyrosine, a neurotransmitter precursor, reduces environmental stress in humans. *Brain Research Bulletin* 22: 759–62.

Beckmann, H., D. Athen, M. Olteanu, and R. Zimmer. 1979. *Archiv fuer Psychiatrie and Nervenkrankheiten* 227: 49–58.

Beckmann, H., M. A. Strauss, and E. Ludolph. 1977. Dl-phenylalanine in depressed patients: An open study. *Journal of Neural Transmission* 41: 123–34.

Benjamin, J., G. Agam, J. Levine, Y. Bersudsky, et al. 1995. Inositol treatment in psychiatry. *Psychopharmocology Bulletin* 31: 167–75.

Benjamin, J., J. Levine, M. Fux, et al. 1995. Double-blind, placebo-controlled, crossover trial of inositol treatment for panic disorder. *American Journal of Psychiatry* 152: 1084–86.

Editor. 1989. Treatment of narcolepsy with tyrosine. *Nutrition Research Newsletter*. February: 18.

Elwes, R. D. C., L. P. Chesterman, P. Jenner, et al. 1989. Treatment of narcolepsy with l-tyrosine: Double-blind placebo controlled trial. *The Lancet* 2: 1067–69.

Fux, M., J. Levine, A. Aviv, and R. H. Belmaker. 1996. Inositol treatment of obsessive-compulsive disorder. *American Journal of Psychiatry* 153: 1219–21.

Gelenberg, A. J., J. D. Wojcik, W. E. Falk, et al. 1990. Tyrosine for depression: A double-blind trial. *Journal of Affective Disorders* 19: 125–32.

Gelenberg, A. J., J. D. Wojcik, C. J. Gibson, and R. J. Wurtman. 1982. Tyrosine for depression. *Journal of Psychiatric Research* 17: 175–80.

Hector, M., and J. R. Burton. 1988. What are the psychiatric manifestations of vitamin B_{12} deficiency? *Journal of the American Geriatrics Society* 36: 1105–12.

Henrotte, J. G. 1986. Type A behavior and magnesium metabolism. *Magnesium* 5: 201–10.

Hutto, B. R. 1997. Folate and cobalamin in psychiatric illness. *Comparative Psychiatry* 38: 305–14.

Levine, J. 1997. Controlled trials of inositol in psychiatry. *European Neuropsychopharmacology* 7: 147–55.

Levine, J., Y. Barak, M. Gonzalves, H. Szor, et al. 1995. Double-blind, controlled trial of inositol treatment of depression. *American Journal of Psychiatry* 152: 792–94.

Maleskey, G. 1989. Battling disease with the amino factor. *Prevention.* May: 61–65.

Owasoyo, J. O., D. F. Neri, and J. G. Lamberth. 1992. *Aviation, Space, and Environmental Medicine* 63:364–69.

Petrie, W. M., and T. A. Tan. 1985. Vitamins in psychiatry. Do they have a role? *Drugs* 30: 58–65.

Taylor, D. S. 1989. Handle stress with diet and supplements. *Better Nutrition.* July: 14–15.

Young, S. N., and A. M. Ghadirian. 1989. *Progress in Neuropsychopharmacology and Biological Psychiatry* 13: 841–63.

CHAPTER FOURTEEN
What You Should Know about Taking Kava: How Much, What Kind, Where to Buy

Almeida, J. C., and E. W. Grimsley. 1996. Coma from the health food store: Interaction between kava and alprazolam. *Annals of Internal Medicine* 125: 940–41.

Cosgrove, J. 1998. The quest for quality. *Nutritional Outlook.* June/July: 22–24, 26.

Duke, J. A. 1997. *The green pharmacy.* Emmaus, Penn.: Rodale Press.

Duve, R. N. 1981. Quality evaluation of yaqona *(Piper methysticum)* in Fiji. *Fiji Agricultural Journal* 43: 1–8.

Hocart, C. H., B. Fankhauser, and David W. Buckle. 1993. Chemical archaeology of kava, a potent brew. *Rapid Communications in Mass Spectrometry* 7: 219–24.

Lebot, V., M. Merlin, and L. Lindstrom. 1997. *Kava: The Pacific Elixir.* New Haven: Yale University Press.

Mayell, M. 1997. Do-it-yourself natural pharmacy. *Natural Health.* March/April: 114–31.

McCormack, S. 1998. Zen in a bottle. *Forbes Magazine.* May 15:46.

Singh, Y. N. 1992. Kava: An overview. *Journal of Ethnopharmacology* 37: 13–45.

APPENDIX A
Kava Questions and Answers

Dolby, V. 1998. Anxiety: Send herbs, 5-htp, and amino acids to the rescue. *Better Nutrition.* June: 18.

Editor. 1998. Getting straight facts on herbs. *Tufts University Health & Nutrition Letter.* May: 1.

Heiligenstein, E., and G. Guenther. 1998. Over-the-counter psychotropics: A review of melatonin, St. John's wort, valerian, and kava-kava. *Journal of American College Health* 46: 271–76.

White, L. B. 1996. No more tossing and turning: Drug-free ways to get your zzz's. *Vegetarian Times*. November: 34–37.

Index